I0429389

A simple, easy to follow programme to help you boost your fitness and get healthy.

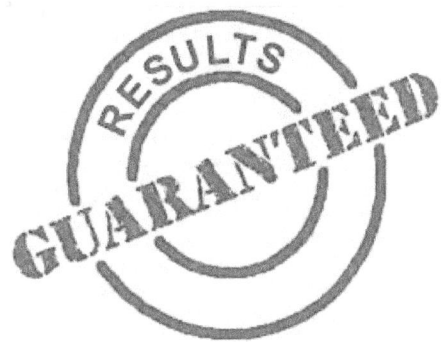

RESULTS GUARANTEED

What have you got to lose?

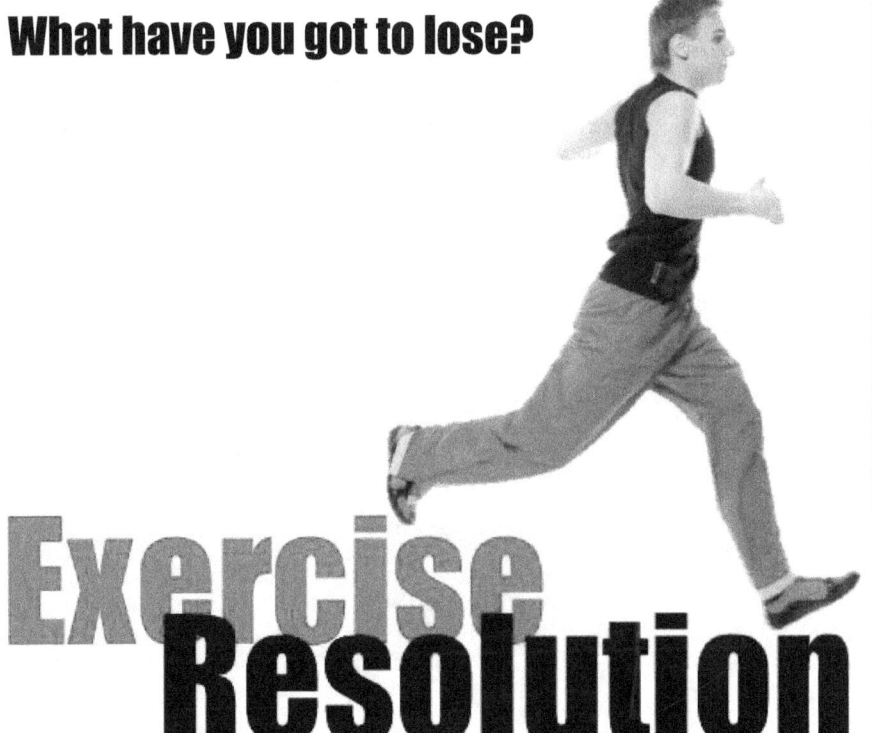

Exercise Resolution

By Andrew Banks

Exercise Resolution

By Andrew Banks

Dedication

This programme is dedicated to my family, Maria, Stacey, Jade and Phoebe for putting up with me during the time I have put in developing this. I know I do not always make it easy. Thank you so much.

Disclaimer

Although we have attempted to make this programme a simple and easy system to follow we do recommend that you always seek the advice of your doctor should you be embarking on this level of exercise for the first time or should you start having any adverse side effects from the exercises you are doing.

Undertaking physical exercise, although good for you, can cause adverse effects on the body if there are any underlying conditions and these should always be checked with a doctor first.

Exercise Resolution

By Andrew Banks

Dear Customer,

Thank you for purchasing the Exercise Resolution programme. By doing so you have already taken the first step towards improving your fitness levels for the next 12 months. This is great for you. I know personally how difficult it can be to get the motivation to carry out something like this. We all live very busy lives with little time to commit to things, but the benefit of this product is that it can be done from the comfort of your own home and will take little time to complete.

All we ask is that you spend between 5—10 minutes a day carrying out these simple steps to help improve and boost your fitness levels. But why is fitness so important? Well I will tell you. Scientifically it has been proven that fitness will help you to:

- increase your energy levels
- feel better about yourself
- maintain personal focus
- keep your body healthy and in shape
- improve your personal efficiency
- reduce the chance of heart disease and other medical problems

These are all great reasons why keeping fit is a great idea. Some may have even considered this as a way to lose some weight. This programme will help you to achieve that. In the end though it will be your hard work that will conquer your personal targets and challenges and I know you can do it.

Stick with it and I can personally guarantee you will see an improvement within the first month.

Remember if you need any support, a pep talk or just some advice on how to progress you can always get in touch. Call or text 07800 957766 and I will personally help you as much as possible.

Regards

Andrew Banks
Creator of Exercise Resolution

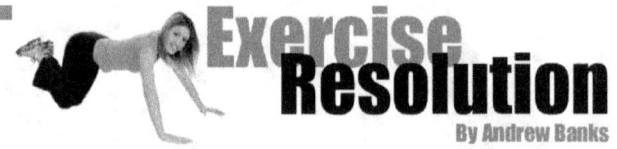

Exercise Resolution
By Andrew Banks

About **You**

Name: _____

Age: _____

Date of Birth: _____/_____/_____

Date Starting: _____/_____/_____

Current Weight (pounds): _____

Current Arm Size (Inches): _____

Current Leg Size (Inches): _____

Current Waist Size (Inches): _____

Current BMI: _____ please see BMI Calculation section for help

I promise to undertake the **Exercise Resolution Programme** and stick to this so that I may feel better about myself once I have started to achieve that which I set out to.

Signed: _____

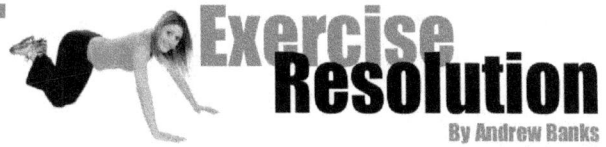

By Andrew Banks

Introduction

Welcome to the Exercise Resolution. A concept that we hope will help you achieve your goal of being fitter and happier. This was developed as there are a lot of people who choose this option as part of their New Year's Resolution but struggle to get the help they need to achieve it without spending hundreds of pounds throughout the year. This is just not necessary and so the Exercise Resolution was born. We will help you to understand what you can and should be doing alongside providing you with the tools you need to monitor your progress.

We have a week by week planner for the first 30 weeks that you can fill out and follow to help you achieve your goals with the option for customisation should you feel you would like to take your training up a notch.

The first thing we will look at is how to follow the programme as well as explanations for the exercises we will be asking you to do. These may seem like standard run of the mill exercises that need no explanation and perhaps you are right, but ask yourself one simple question, are you doing them at the moment?

We need to ensure that you know what you are doing first and foremost before we ask you to carry these out on a daily basis. This is to prevent injury and the development of bad habits.

So, without further ado let's look at the Exercise Resolution.

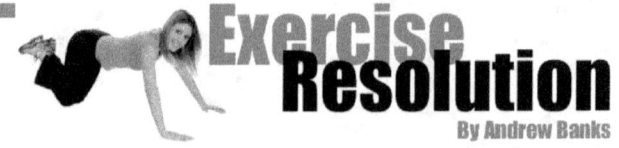

By Andrew Banks

Monitoring

We have provided you with a series of monitoring sheets that you can fill out on a weekly basis to help you track your progress for the first 30 weeks. These have been designed to make this an easy system for you to follow.

We not only help you keep a log of the exercises that you have done in a tick sheet format but we also help you to monitor certain areas of your body such as weight, waist size and your BMI (Body Mass Index). These we will cover in more depth later on.

If, for whatever reason, you cannot keep up with the amounts specified, this is also ok. The fact is everyone is different and therefore we have allowed customisation of the programme. You will find a custom monitoring sheet available too that will enable you to put in your own targets that you have set yourself. This can be photocopied so that you have access to more than one. You can also download them at any time from: http://goo.gl/VF1N5

Taking part in this programme is not a race against time. You have all the time you can allow yourself to achieve the targets that we have set as well as your own.

Calculating

When it comes to filling out your monitoring sheets you have a series of tick boxes. All this requires is for you to tick once you have completed each exercise. Once you have finished the week you will just total up how many of each you have achieved. This will help you to see how much in a week you have actually completed. This can be a running total for you to look at and see just how well you are doing.

Once you have finished each day you will have the second side of the sheet to fill in also. This should be done either before you start the exercises or after, but whichever you decide to do you must continue to do so throughout the programme. This ensures that the information on the sheets

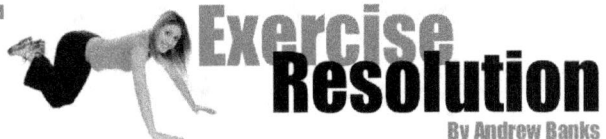
is accurate and fair in comparison.

Each section should be completed where possible so that you can get a bigger picture as to your progress. Depending on your current physical condition, you may not see differences in size but you may in muscle tone. Some people keep video or photo diaries to accompany their progress. This is your choice but at least ensure you pay attention to how your body changes.

We also need certain measurements for each section. If you need to convert these from what your scales and tape measures provide this is not a problem.

Weight

Most people have scales that will tell you how much you weigh in stone and pounds or Kilos. No matter which you have you will need to do a conversion to put the information onto your sheets so that it is easier to work out your BMI.

Stone and Pounds → Pounds

There are 14lbs to a Stone so use this calculation

Weight from Scales: ____Stone ____lbs.

$$\underline{\hspace{3cm}} \textbf{ x 14} + \underline{\hspace{3cm}} = \underline{\hspace{2cm}}\textbf{lbs.}$$
Stone Amount   **lbs Amount**

Kilos → Pounds

There are approximately 2.2lbs to every Kilogram so use this calculation

$$\underline{\hspace{3cm}} \textbf{÷2.2} = \underline{\hspace{2cm}}\textbf{lbs.}$$
Kilos Amount

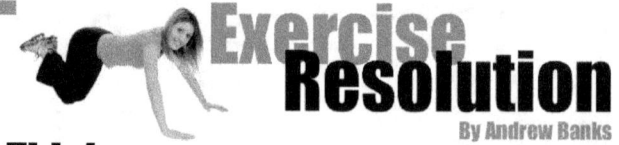

Exercise Resolution

By Andrew Banks

Waist, Arms and Thighs

We ask that while you are carrying out the programme that you also monitor your Waist, Arm and Thigh sizes throughout. This will probably be most important for those who are looking to lose weight but it is just another area in which you can see progress as well.

Checking the Waist

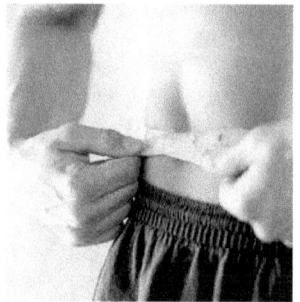

To check the measurement for your waist you simple wrap the tape measure around your body keeping the tape measure in line with navel or just below. You can then record this onto your monitoring sheet.

Checking the Arms

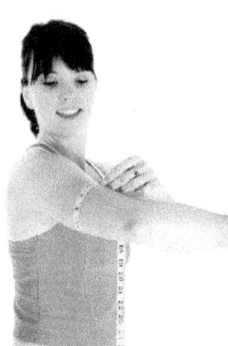

When checking the measurement of the arms we ask that you pick one side to keep track on but obviously you can measure both. Simply wrap the tape measure around the middle of the upper arm and take the measurement in Inches. You can then record this on your monitoring sheet.

Checking the Thighs

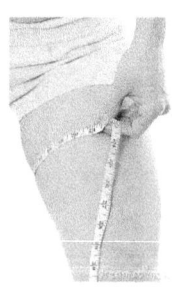

When it comes to measuring the thighs, this works in the same way as checking the arms. You will pick one thigh that you will monitor but you can take the measurements off of both. Wrap the tape measure around the middle of the thigh and record the measurement on the monitoring sheet.

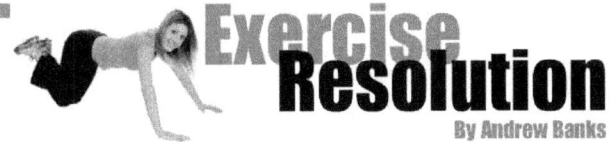

By Andrew Banks

When measuring your arms and your thighs you may have a tape measure that works n centimetres and not inches. That is ok; a simple conversion will help that.

_____ **x 0.39 = _____lbs.**
CM Amount

BMI Calculation

Your BMI, otherwise known as a Body Mass Index, is a scale used to determine whether your body is overweight or not. Now please do not assume for one moment that this is 100% accurate as in the end everybody is different. This does however give you an indication and has been used by medical professionals for years. Now there are several levels that BMI categorise. These are:

BMI	Weight Status
Below 18.5	Underweight
18.5 – 24.9	Normal
25 – 29.9	Overweight
30 and above	Obese

When completing your monitoring sheets you will need to calculate your BMI to see what category you fit into. This is done using a simple calculation. However if you prefer to use an online calculator please feel free to visit: http://www.bmicalculator.co.uk/

For those who are happy to carry out the calculation the old fashioned way here is the math.

Firstly we need to know your height in inches. Most people know their height in feet and inches so we need to convert this first.

_____ **x 12 + _____ = _____Inches**
Foot Amount   **Inch Amount**

The calculation for BMI is as follows

$$BMI = \frac{(\text{Weight in pounds x 703})}{(\text{Height in Inches x Height in Inches})}$$

We will break that into stages to make is a little easier.

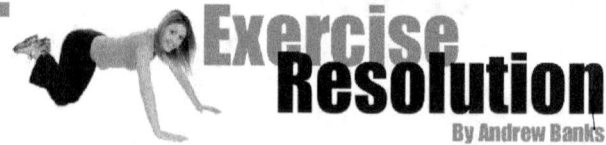

Exercise Resolution
By Andrew Banks

Stage 1

_____ x 703 = _____ Stage 1 Answer
Weight in lbs.

Stage 2

_____ X _____ = _____ Stage 2 Answer
Height in   Height in
Inches   Inches

Stage 3

_____ ÷ _____ = _____ Your BMI
Stage 1 Answer   Stage 2 Answer

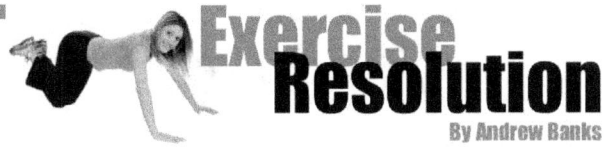

Exercise Resolution

By Andrew Banks

Eating

Unlike other fitness strategies that exist we will not be detailing what food you can and cannot eat. What we will do is help you to understand your daily limits and help you understand some fundamental rules that are often missed out.

The fact is that many diet plans that exist today explain how you can get the body you want just by adjusting your diet. The problem with this is that they will either not work or they will only work short term because in order for your body to become fit and healthy it will require a lifestyle change. Half the time the diets of people who go on these diet plans are actually ok, the problem ends up being that they have no counter balance to their diet.

As you can see from the diagrams below it is important to have a good balance between eating and exercise.

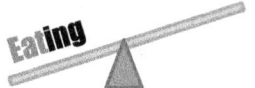
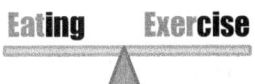
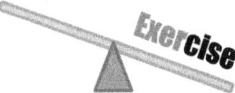

If you only eat with little to no exercise then your weight will go up. This will drastically reduce your health.

If you eat and exercise in moderation then your weight will stay around the same size if in balance with each other.

If you do a lot of exercise but do not eat enough or not in proportion then your weight will fall faster. This will drastically reduce your health.

Your body works based on your metabolism, its designed to process your food and turn it into energy and fat storage. You may well have heard the term that you should eat 3 meals a day? This is not far from the truth. Have you also heard the saying breakfast is the most important meal of the day? Also not far from the truth. The fact is, your body, although great at what it does, still needs some input from you. With this in mind we need to get you to alter your mind set. When carrying out this programme, in order to get the best possible results we would like you to stick to a 3 meal a day routine with the possible 1 off snack. We literally mean snack here and not another full blown meal.

Depending on the area in which you live you will be having:

Breakfast → Lunch → Dinner   Or   **Breakfast → Dinner → Tea**

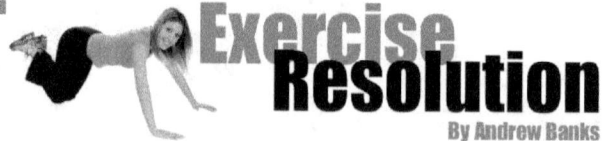

Exercise Resolution

By Andrew Banks

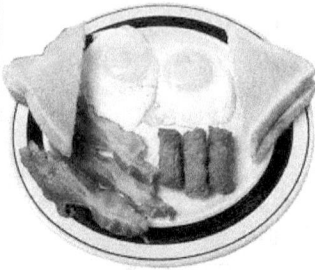

We would like you to stick to these three meals. I know that many of you in todays busy world will skip meals due to schedules etc but this has to stop as it is a very unhealthy thing to do. Many may shy away from eating breakfast as it makes people feel sick or unwell after doing so. This is usually due to your body not knowing how to handle food so early but this is something you need to retrain your body in doing. If you are used to skipping meals start with something small when bringing them back into play. This will be difficult to start with but will not take long for your body to readjust to.

All three meals should be spread throughout the day. Breakfast should be eaten almost as soon as you have woken up with Dinner or Lunch at the mid point of your day with your final meal being at the end of your day with a few hours allowed afterwards for food to settle and start the digestion process. Many people recommend that eating after 8pm is a bad idea as this will sit in your digestive system and not fully digest whilst you sleep.

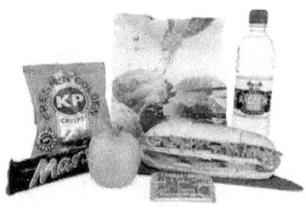

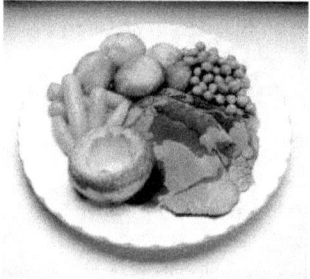

Also keep your portions in moderation. There are recommended daily allowances on calories etc but we are not going to worry you with those as everyone is different as we have explained before and we are not going to stereotype you. Eating food should be down to how much you need. When you have eaten enough to feel full you should stop eating. A lot of people will continue to eat due to still having food left. How many of you have said "I feel really full now" or "maybe I shouldn't have eaten that too"

This is your body telling you that you have eaten more than you should and therefore should slow down. If you know the amount you usually eat is too much, just cut down a little at a time and reduce your portions slowly. Again please remember that this is not a race and you will get there as soon as you can.

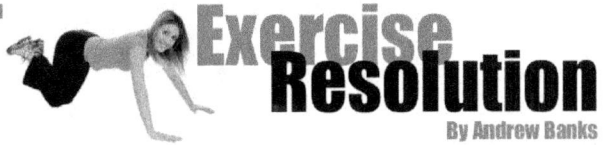

Your Exercises

Ok so now we will look at the exercises we have in store for you to carry out as part of your programme. We understand that you may not like some of these, but at the same time the ones you do not like are probably the ones you need to do more of. Each one will help different areas of the body and will help boost your fitness and health slowly and even better, will cost nothing but a little of your time. No gym fee, just you and your home.

Push Ups

There are two types that we will look at. For some neither will be easy but we still categorise these as beginner and advanced according to their level of difficulty. A push up is a good way to work the muscles in the arms.

Advanced Push Ups

Push Ups should be started with your body being held off the floor by your hands and toes. Your feet should be together with your hands flat on the floor spead shoulder width apart inline with your shoulders. Your back should be straight.

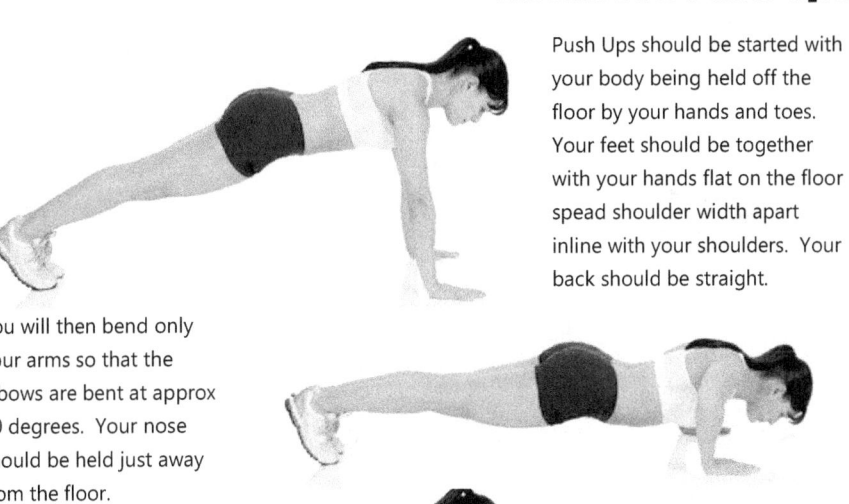

You will then bend only your arms so that the elbows are bent at approx 90 degrees. Your nose should be held just away from the floor.

From here you will then push back up again to the starting position. This will count as one full Push Up.

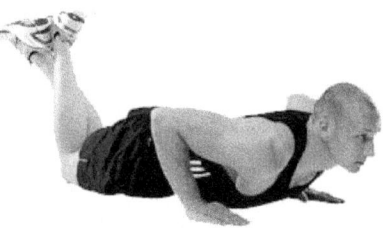

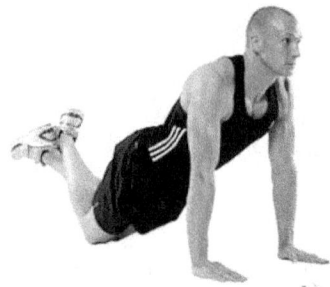

These push ups are exactly the same except the body is held up using the hands and the knees. The feet can be crossed if you so wish but this is not necessary. The back must remain in a straight line as previously stated with the hands shoulder width and inline with shoulders themselves.

As with the advanced method, only the elbows will bend to approximately a 90 degree angle. The nose should not touch the floor.

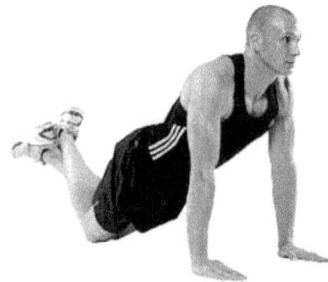

Finally you will push your arms straight again raising your body up back into the starting position. This will be considered a full Push Up.

Sit Ups

As with the Push Ups, Sit Ups have an easy method and a hard method. These are all part of the same process so we will not have to break them down. People make a lot of common mistakes when doing Sit Ups, hopefully we will help you to eliminate these before you start.

Stage 1

Your body needs to be in the right position. This is not just for comfort but also for body safety. You must be laid

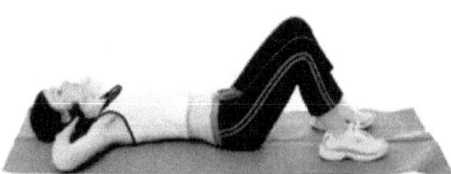

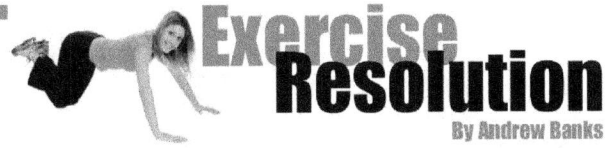

Exercise Resolution
By Andrew Banks

down on the floor firstly. Now an important part to remember is that when you have laid on the floor you are not naturally flat. Your back arches and this can cause problems in later life if you ignore this now so we need to alleviate that. Firstly you will bend your knees and place your feet on the floor spread shoulder width apart. You should then raise your chin to your chest supporting your head by placing your hands behind it. This is your starting position.

Stage 2

From your starting position you will need to use your stomach muscles to pull your body up. You will bring your head and shoulders off of the floor. This is the most that is expected for a beginner as stomach muscles may not be strong 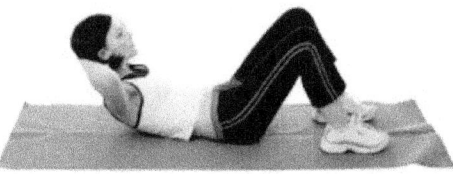 enough to go further yet. This will just take some time to develop. Common mistakes that people make at this stage is to either raise their feet from the floor to generate momentum or remove their hands from the head and grab something to assist. This is a bad thing to do and defeats the object of the exercise. All those using this easy method will now skip to Stage 4. Those who are opting for the harder method will continue to Stage 3.

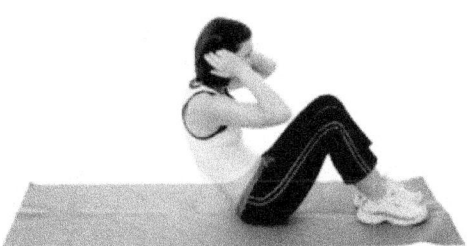

Stage 3

Once you have achieved Stage 2 you will reach a point where you must pull hard using your stomach muscles to pull your body up so that your elbows can touch your knees. Remember, no bad habits. Keep your feet firmly on the floor and your hands behind your head.

Stage 4

Now slowly guide yourself down to the starting position and relax if you have finished your repetitions. That will be considered one whole Push Up.

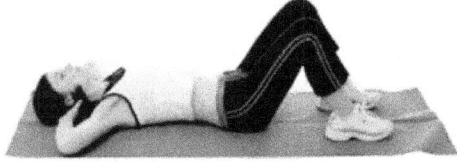

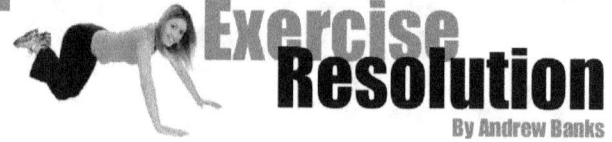

Star Jumps

Star Jumps, or Jumping Jacks depending on where you are from are a great way of getting your arms and legs working together and believe it or not are a great way to improve body co-ordination too.

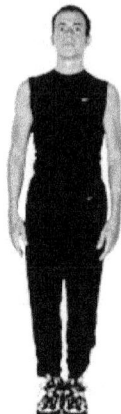

You will start standing up straight with your arms by your side and legs together. This is a nice stationary and almost natural position.

The next step is to simultaniously jump your legs to just beyond shoulder widths apart and pull your arms up in the air so that you look like a star.

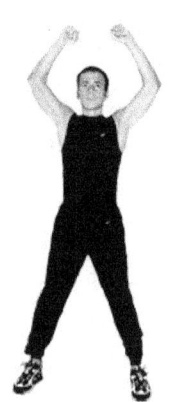

Finally you will again jump simultaniously pulling your arms and legs back to the starting position. This will constitute a single Star Jump

Due to the simplicity of these the rep amount is much higher as it takes less effort than some of the other exercises you will do.

Squat Thrusts

This exercise is a variation on the Push Ups that we have looked at already. These however will require you to support the body using the arms whilst utilising the leg muscles which makes this a great exercise to use.

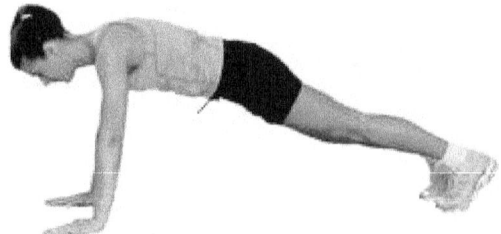

You will start from the main Push Up position where you are supporting your body weight with your hands and legs ensuring that your back is straight.

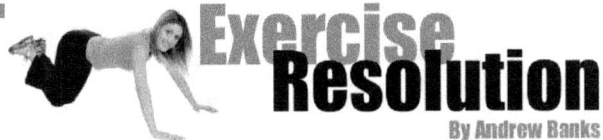

You will then thrust your legs forward whilst keeping your hands in place. You should aim to land your toes so that your knees are bent approximately 90 degrees. This will put your into a squatting position.

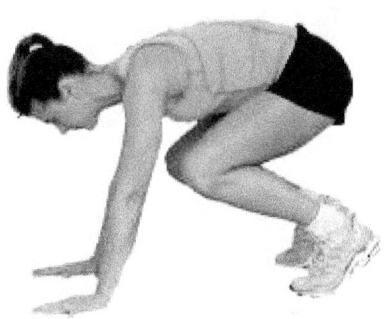

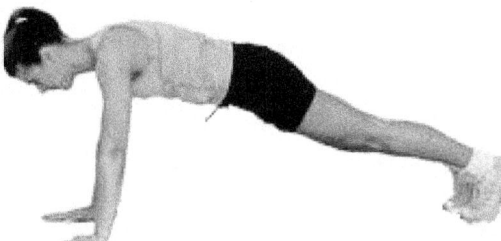

You will then thrust your legs back again to the starting position, ensuring that your back is straight. This will constitute a single Squat Thrust.

Step Ups

With the Step Ups there are two ways in which you can do these. If you already have an exercise step that you can use then great, if not please DO NOT go and buy one. Most of you will have a set of stairs that you can use. You only need one. If you live in a bungalow and do not have a step you can use, maybe you have a step ladder that could work for you. There is always an option without having to spend any more money.

With this one you will start standing straight in front of the step. Then simply place either your left or right foot onto the step.

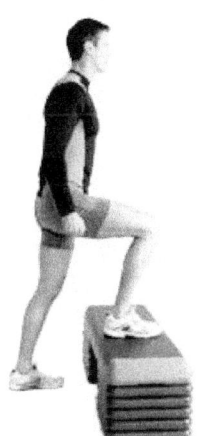

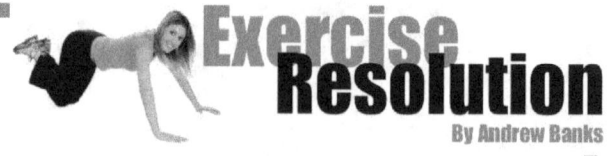

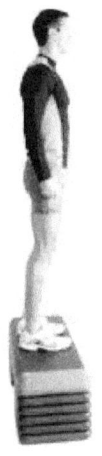

You will then pull your back leg from the floor onto the step.

Then take the leg you started with and place that back down on to the floor, finally bringing your front leg back down to your starting position.

This will constitute a full Step Up.

Should you wish to use a full set of stairs with one foot per step you must double the figure on the monitoing sheet.

Run / Jog

Running and Jogging is something that needs little explanation, however we did want to explain that we do not specify which we would like you to do. This is your choice. You will also notice that the length of time we have specified is very small. This is due to understanding that Runnig and Jogging has been proven that over time causes impact damage on your joints and we would like this to be something you do in moderation as to not cause any problems physically throughout the programme. If you choose to increase your times more then this will be your choice but please remember to moderate everything and not overdo it.

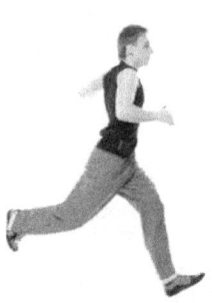

When it comes to the Running or Jogging section, remember that you do not need to go anywhere if you do not wish to. Running on the spot will still be just as good. However, if you can get outside and enjoy the fresh air that comes with it, even better.

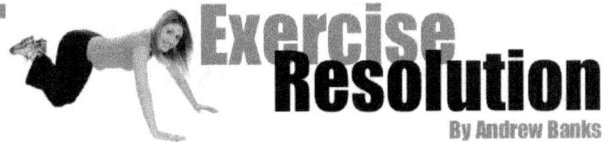

The Aftermath

When you have carried out these exercises there may be a period where you could feel sore or tender. This is not unexpected, especially for those of you who are new to this kind of physical activity. You are getting your muscles to work and in some cases in ways you have not for a while, if ever. This takes some adjustment for your body. Aching and soreness is just your body's way of letting you know that it has taken note of what you want it to do.

If you ever feel like this please just keep going as normal. The worst you can do is stop, this will make your musclles start to revert and therefore you will end up at the beginning. By just carrying on with your daily life you will notice that the feeling can be shurgged off and will stop in a very short space of time.

Hot baths or showers are also a great way to help relieve the pressure from sore and aching muscles so maybe incorporate one of these into your routine everyday.

Please also understand that there is a very distinct difference between soreness or aching and pain. Pain is something that hurts and will not stop. This is due to an actual problem. Should you ever experience pain that does not subside, please contact your Doctor asap. It is always better to be safe than sorry.

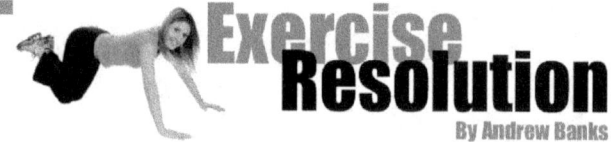

Where?

So where abouts should you carry out your exercises? Well this is up to you in the end. If you prefer the security of your bedroom away from prying eyes or if maybe your front room is the best place then that is fine also. You need to find a place that will allow you space and freedom of movement. Some people even prefer to have a music channel on in the background so that they have a beat to work with. It is whatever you need and choose to make this the best experience it can be for you.

Targets and Milestones

Througout the programme you will notice that we have give you some milestones and targets to achieve and accomplish. However we can only guide you so far. It is important in life to be able to set your own goals and targets so we also allow for that too. The custom monitoring sheets are designed to allow you to do just that. If you prefer your own targets from the start or if you would like to go above and beyond what we have outlined then please do. This is your programme and you should be able to customise it if you see fit.

Let's have a look at the milestones we have set for you so far though.

	Target 1	Target 2	Target 3	Target 4	Target 5
Push Ups	10	20	30	40	50
Sit Ups	10	20	30	40	50
Star Jumps	30	40	50		
Squat Thrusts	10	20	30	40	50
Step Ups	30	40	50		
Run / Jog Ups	2 mins	3mins	4 mins	5 mins	

Although we have provided you with pre-determined monitoring guides for the first 30 weeks to help you get to each milestone, these are only guides. A guideline on what we feel would be good progress, but remember, anything is good progress just stick with it.

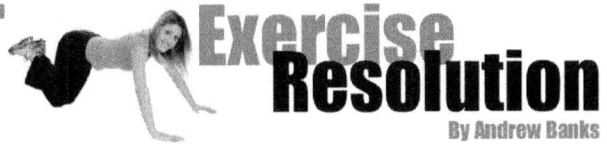

By Andrew Banks

You may want to push your limitations and achieve 100 of each exercise with a 30 minute run or jog. This is completely your choice.

If you ever feel like it is getting hard, or you ever feel like maybe not doing it for one day follow this simple flow chart

Should I Workout Today?

Yes

No

Go workout

Yes you should

The fact is, if you stop, it is hard to start again. This programme needs to be taken seriously from the word go. Just keep telling yourself, You Can Do This!

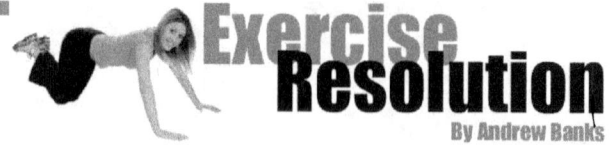

After Week 30?

This is a dreaded way point, when the decisions start becoming your own and you may feel a little worried or anxious over how you should proceed. This is because you are taking steps into unfamiliar territory. But at the same time it is still familiar. The exercises you are doing are still the same, you just need to make your own targets and go from there.

We have even supplied a target sheet for you to fill in to give yourself a set of targets from week 30 onwards.

When you set your targets, remember to make them SMART. Specific, Measurable, Attainable, Relevant and finally Timebound, that way you can see how well you are achieving your goals.

What about when I finish 52 weeks?

In theory you will never truly finish as this should be an ongoing cycle. But once you reach week 52 get in touch with us. We will assess your progress and we will then send you a certificate to congratulate you on your achievement.

What Now?

Now all you need to do is set a start date. Make sure you start on a Monday, it is a fresh week so you can start all in one go. Also remember that Sunday is your day of rest, even when you exercise you should have one. The rest is up to you. If you need any help please contact us or even check out the facebook page. Just search "Exercise Resolution" and discuss your findings or seek any assistance you need.

Good luck with the programme and remember **YOU CAN DO IT!!!**

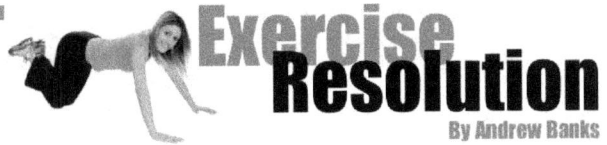

Notes

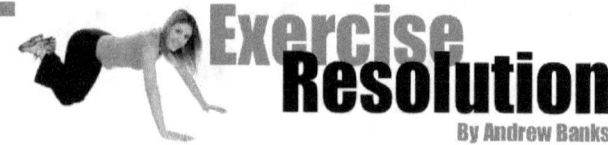

Notes

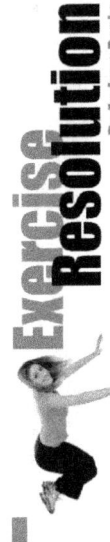

Exercise Resolution

By Andrew Banks

Progress Chart—Week 1

Exercise	Monday Required	Monday Complete?	Tuesday Required	Tuesday Complete?	Wednesday Required	Wednesday Complete?	Thursday Required	Thursday Complete?	Friday Required	Friday Complete?	Saturday Required	Saturday Complete?	Total
Push Ups	5	☐	5	☐	6	☐	6	☐	8	☐	8	☐	
Sit Ups	5	☐	5	☐	6	☐	6	☐	8	☐	8	☐	
Star Jumps	10	☐	10	☐	12	☐	12	☐	12	☐	15	☐	
Squat Thrusts	5	☐	5	☐	6	☐	6	☐	8	☐	8	☐	
Step Ups	20	☐	20	☐	20	☐	20	☐	20	☐	20	☐	
Run / Jog	-	☐	-	☐	-	☐	-	☐	-	☐	-	☐	

Exercise Resolution
By Andrew Banks

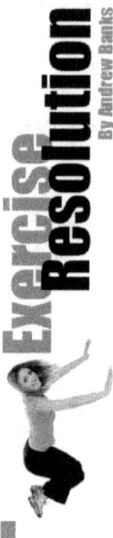

Progress Chart—Week 1

Personal Stats	Monday		Tuesday		Wednesday		Thursday		Friday		Saturday	
	Current	Up or Down	Current	Up or Down	Current	Up or Down	Current	Up or Down	Current	Up or Down	Current	Up or Down
Weight (Pounds)												
Waist Size (Inches)												
Arm Size (Inches)												
Thigh Size (Inches)												
BMI												

BMI Calculation

$$BMI = \frac{(\text{Weight in pounds} \times 703)}{(\text{Height in Inches} \times \text{Height in Inches})}$$

If you are unsure about working out any of these statistics then please refer to the main guide book which will explain these to you in more detail and help you to understand it better. Remember, you are doing well, keep it up.

Exercise Resolution
By Andrew Banks

Progress Chart—Week 10

Exercise	Monday Required	Monday Complete?	Tuesday Required	Tuesday Complete?	Wednesday Required	Wednesday Complete?	Thursday Required	Thursday Complete?	Friday Required	Friday Complete?	Saturday Required	Saturday Complete?	Total
Push Ups	10	☐	10	☐	10	☐	10	☐	10	☐	10	☐	
Sit Ups	10	☐	10	☐	10	☐	10	☐	10	☐	10	☐	
Star Jumps	30	☐	30	☐	30	☐	30	☐	30	☐	30	☐	
Squat Thrusts	10	☐	10	☐	10	☐	10	☐	10	☐	10	☐	
Step Ups	30	☐	30	☐	30	☐	30	☐	30	☐	30	☐	
Run / Jog	2 mins	☐	2 mins	☐	2 mins	☐	2 mins	☐	2 mins	☐	2 mins	☐	

Exercise Resolution
By Andrew Banks

Progress Chart—Week 10

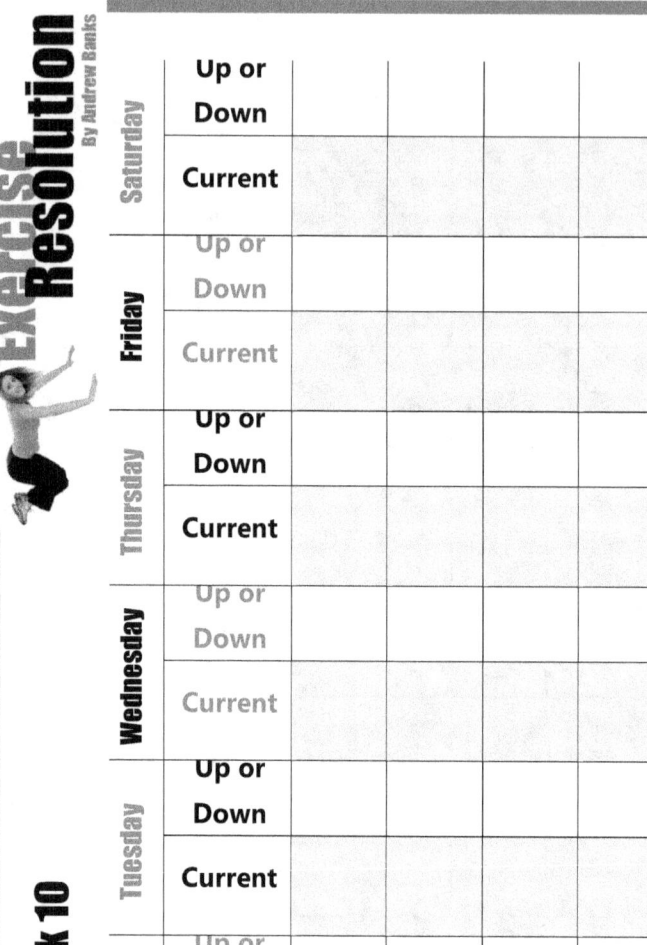

Personal Stats	Monday Current	Monday Up or Down	Tuesday Current	Tuesday Up or Down	Wednesday Current	Wednesday Up or Down	Thursday Current	Thursday Up or Down	Friday Current	Friday Up or Down	Saturday Current	Saturday Up or Down
Weight (Pounds)												
Waist Size (Inches)												
Arm Size (Inches)												
Thigh Size (Inches)												
BMI												

BMI Calculation

$$BMI = \frac{(\text{Weight in pounds} \times 703)}{(\text{Height in Inches} \times \text{Height in Inches})}$$

If you are unsure about working out any of these statistics then please refer to the main guide book which will explain these to you in more detail and help you to understand it better. Remember, you are doing well, keep it up.

Exercise Resolution
By Andrew Banks

Progress Chart—Week 11

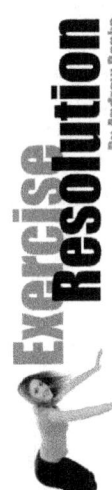

Exercise	Monday Required	Monday Complete?	Tuesday Required	Tuesday Complete?	Wednesday Required	Wednesday Complete?	Thursday Required	Thursday Complete?	Friday Required	Friday Complete?	Saturday Required	Saturday Complete?	Total
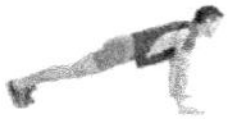 Push Ups	10	☐	10	☐	12	☐	12	☐	14	☐	14	☐	
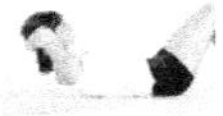 Sit Ups	10	☐	10	☐	12	☐	12	☐	14	☐	14	☐	
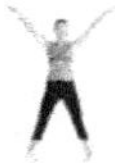 Star Jumps	30	☐	30	☐	34	☐	34	☐	36	☐	36	☐	
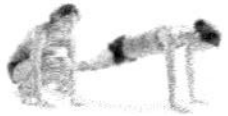 Squat Thrusts	10	☐	10	☐	12	☐	12	☐	14	☐	14	☐	
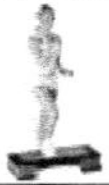 Step Ups	30	☐	30	☐	34	☐	34	☐	36	☐	36	☐	
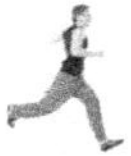 Run / Jog	2 mins	☐	2 mins	☐	2 mins	☐	2 mins	☐	2 mins	☐	2 mins	☐	

Exercise Resolution
By Andrew Banks

Progress Chart—Week 11

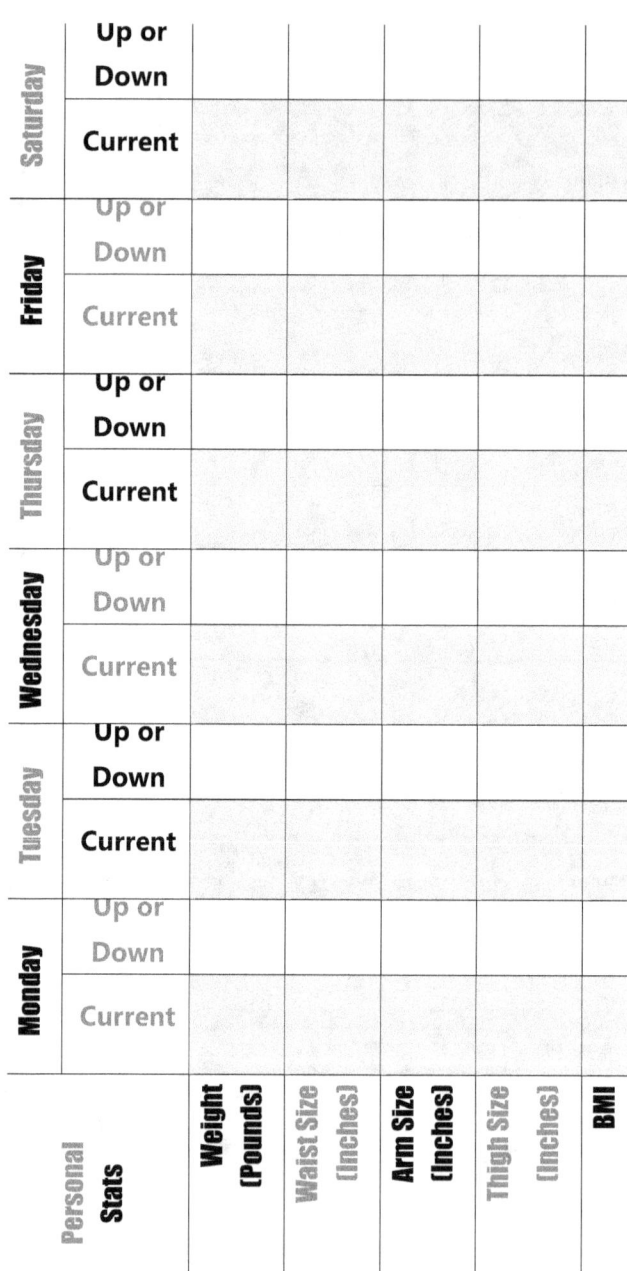

Personal Stats	Monday		Tuesday		Wednesday		Thursday		Friday		Saturday	
	Current	Up or Down	Current	Up or Down	Current	Up or Down	Current	Up or Down	Current	Up or Down	Current	Up or Down
Weight (Pounds)												
Waist Size (Inches)												
Arm Size (Inches)												
Thigh Size (Inches)												
BMI												

BMI Calculation

$$BMI = \frac{(\text{Weight in pounds} \times 703)}{(\text{Height in Inches} \times \text{Height in Inches})}$$

If you are unsure about working out any of these statistics then please refer to the main guide book which will explain these to you in more detail and help you to understand it better. Remember, you are doing well, keep it up.

Exercise Resolution
By Andrew Banks

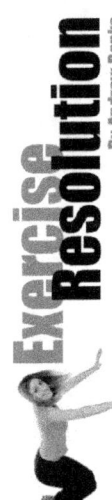

Progress Chart—Week 12

Exercise	Monday Required	Monday Complete?	Tuesday Required	Tuesday Complete?	Wednesday Required	Wednesday Complete?	Thursday Required	Thursday Complete?	Friday Required	Friday Complete?	Saturday Required	Saturday Complete?	Total
Push Ups	10	☐	10	☐	12	☐	12	☐	14	☐	14	☐	
Sit Ups	10	☐	10	☐	12	☐	12	☐	14	☐	14	☐	
Star Jumps	30	☐	30	☐	34	☐	34	☐	36	☐	36	☐	
Squat Thrusts	10	☐	10	☐	12	☐	12	☐	14	☐	14	☐	
Step Ups	30	☐	30	☐	34	☐	34	☐	36	☐	36	☐	
Run / Jog	3 mins	☐	3 mins	☐	3 mins	☐	3 mins	☐	3 mins	☐	3 mins	☐	

Exercise Resolution
By Andrew Banks

Progress Chart—Week 12

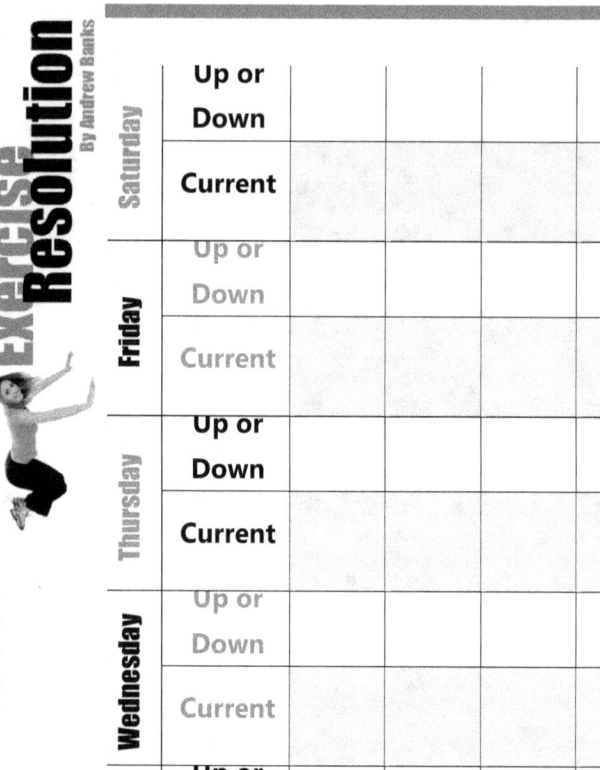

Personal Stats	Monday		Tuesday		Wednesday		Thursday		Friday		Saturday	
	Current	Up or Down	Current	Up or Down	Current	Up or Down	Current	Up or Down	Current	Up or Down	Current	Up or Down
Weight (Pounds)												
Waist Size (Inches)												
Arm Size (Inches)												
Thigh Size (Inches)												
BMI												

BMI Calculation

$$BMI = \frac{(\text{Weight in pounds} \times 703)}{(\text{Height in Inches} \times \text{Height in Inches})}$$

If you are unsure about working out any of these statistics then please refer to the main guide book which will explain these to you in more detail and help you to understand it better. Remember, you are doing well, keep it up.

Exercise Resolution
By Andrew Banks

Progress Chart—Week 13

Exercise	Monday Required	Monday Complete?	Tuesday Required	Tuesday Complete?	Wednesday Required	Wednesday Complete?	Thursday Required	Thursday Complete?	Friday Required	Friday Complete?	Saturday Required	Saturday Complete?	Total
Push Ups	12	☐	12	☐	14	☐	14	☐	16	☐	16	☐	
Sit Ups	12	☐	12	☐	14	☐	14	☐	16	☐	16	☐	
Star Jumps	34	☐	34	☐	36	☐	36	☐	38	☐	38	☐	
Squat Thrusts	12	☐	12	☐	14	☐	14	☐	16	☐	16	☐	
Step Ups	34	☐	34	☐	36	☐	36	☐	38	☐	38	☐	
Run / Jog	3 mins	☐	3 mins	☐	3 mins	☐	3 mins	☐	3 mins	☐	3 mins	☐	

Exercise Resolution
By Andrew Banks

Progress Chart—Week 13

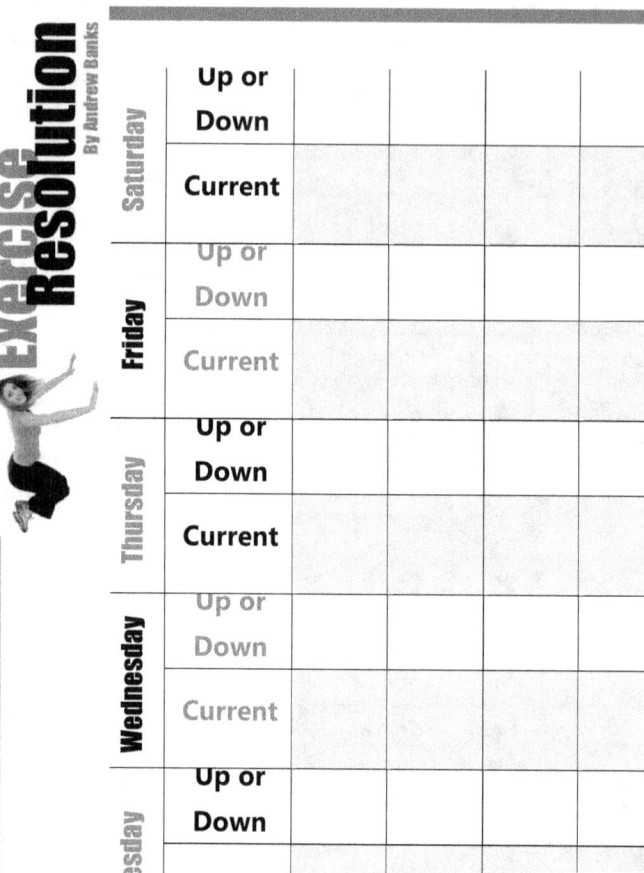

Personal Stats	Monday		Tuesday		Wednesday		Thursday		Friday		Saturday	
	Current	Up or Down	Current	Up or Down	Current	Up or Down	Current	Up or Down	Current	Up or Down	Current	Up or Down
Weight (Pounds)												
Waist Size (Inches)												
Arm Size (Inches)												
Thigh Size (Inches)												
BMI												

BMI Calculation

$$BMI = \frac{(Weight\ in\ pounds \times 703)}{(Height\ in\ Inches \times Height\ in\ Inches)}$$

If you are unsure about working out any of these statistics then please refer to the main guide book which will explain these to you in more detail and help you to understand it better. Remember, you are doing well, keep it up.

Exercise Resolution
By Andrew Banks

Progress Chart—Week 14

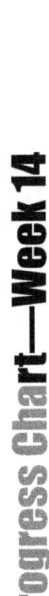

Exercise	Monday Required	Monday Complete?	Tuesday Required	Tuesday Complete?	Wednesday Required	Wednesday Complete?	Thursday Required	Thursday Complete?	Friday Required	Friday Complete?	Saturday Required	Saturday Complete?	Total
Push Ups	14	☐	14	☐	16	☐	16	☐	18	☐	18	☐	
Sit Ups	14	☐	14	☐	16	☐	16	☐	18	☐	18	☐	
Star Jumps	36	☐	36	☐	38	☐	38	☐	40	☐	40	☐	
Squat Thrusts	14	☐	14	☐	16	☐	16	☐	18	☐	18	☐	
Step Ups	36	☐	36	☐	38	☐	38	☐	40	☐	40	☐	
Run / Jog	3 mins	☐	3 mins	☐	3 mins	☐	3 mins	☐	3 mins	☐	3 mins	☐	

Exercise Resolution
By Andrew Banks

Progress Chart—Week 14

Personal Stats	Monday		Tuesday		Wednesday		Thursday		Friday		Saturday	
	Current	Up or Down	Current	Up or Down	Current	Up or Down	Current	Up or Down	Current	Up or Down	Current	Up or Down
Weight [Pounds]												
Waist Size [Inches]												
Arm Size [Inches]												
Thigh Size [Inches]												
BMI												

BMI Calculation

$$BMI = \frac{(Weight\ in\ pounds \times 703\ )}{(Height\ in\ Inches \times Height\ in\ Inches)}$$

If you are unsure about working out any of these statistics then please refer to the main guide book which will explain these to you in more detail and help you to understand it better. Remember, you are doing well, keep it up.

Exercise Resolution
By Andrew Banks

Progress Chart—Week 15

Exercise	Monday Required	Monday Complete?	Tuesday Required	Tuesday Complete?	Wednesday Required	Wednesday Complete?	Thursday Required	Thursday Complete?	Friday Required	Friday Complete?	Saturday Required	Saturday Complete?	Total
Push Ups	16	☐	16	☐	18	☐	18	☐	20	☐	20	☐	
Sit Ups	16	☐	16	☐	18	☐	18	☐	20	☐	20	☐	
Star Jumps	38	☐	38	☐	40	☐	40	☐	40	☐	40	☐	
Squat Thrusts	16	☐	16	☐	18	☐	18	☐	20	☐	20	☐	
Step Ups	38	☐	38	☐	40	☐	40	☐	40	☐	40	☐	
Run / Jog	3 mins	☐	3 mins	☐	3 mins	☐	3 mins	☐	3 mins	☐	3 mins	☐	

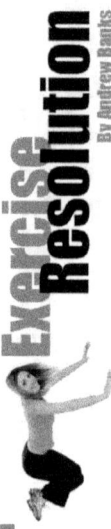

Exercise Resolution
By Andrew Banks

Progress Chart—Week 15

Personal Stats	Monday		Tuesday		Wednesday		Thursday		Friday		Saturday	
	Current	Up or Down	Current	Up or Down	Current	Up or Down	Current	Up or Down	Current	Up or Down	Current	Up or Down
Weight (Pounds)												
Waist Size (Inches)												
Arm Size (Inches)												
Thigh Size (Inches)												
BMI												

BMI Calculation

$$BMI = \frac{(\text{Weight in pounds} \times 703\,)}{(\text{Height in Inches} \times \text{Height in Inches})}$$

If you are unsure about working out any of these statistics then please refer to the main guide book which will explain these to you in more detail and help you to understand it better. Remember, you are doing well, keep it up.

Exercise Resolution
By Andrew Banks

Progress Chart—Week 16

Exercise		Monday Required	Monday Complete?	Tuesday Required	Tuesday Complete?	Wednesday Required	Wednesday Complete?	Thursday Required	Thursday Complete?	Friday Required	Friday Complete?	Saturday Required	Saturday Complete?	Total
Push Ups	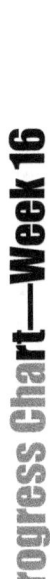	18	☐	18	☐	20	☐	20	☐	20	☐	20	☐	
Sit Ups		18	☐	18	☐	20	☐	20	☐	20	☐	20	☐	
Star Jumps		40	☐	40	☐	40	☐	40	☐	40	☐	40	☐	
Squat Thrusts		18	☐	18	☐	20	☐	20	☐	20	☐	20	☐	
Step Ups		40	☐	40	☐	40	☐	40	☐	40	☐	40	☐	
Run / Jog		3 mins	☐	3 mins	☐	3 mins	☐	3 mins	☐	3 mins	☐	3 mins	☐	

Exercise Resolution
By Andrew Banks

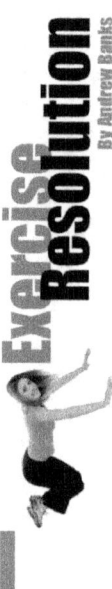

Progress Chart—Week 16

Personal Stats	Monday		Tuesday		Wednesday		Thursday		Friday		Saturday	
	Current	Up or Down	Current	Up or Down	Current	Up or Down	Current	Up or Down	Current	Up or Down	Current	Up or Down
Weight [Pounds]												
Waist Size [Inches]												
Arm Size [Inches]												
Thigh Size [Inches]												
BMI												

BMI Calculation

$$BMI = \frac{(\text{Weight in pounds} \times 703)}{(\text{Height in Inches} \times \text{Height in Inches})}$$

If you are unsure about working out any of these statistics then please refer to the main guide book which will explain these to you in more detail and help you to understand it better. Remember, you are doing well, keep it up.

Exercise Resolution
By Andrew Banks

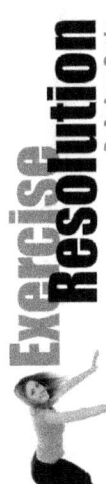

Progress Chart—Week 17

Exercise	Monday Required	Monday Complete?	Tuesday Required	Tuesday Complete?	Wednesday Required	Wednesday Complete?	Thursday Required	Thursday Complete?	Friday Required	Friday Complete?	Saturday Required	Saturday Complete?	Total
Push Ups	20	☐	20	☐	20	☐	20	☐	20	☐	20	☐	
Sit Ups	20	☐	20	☐	20	☐	20	☐	20	☐	20	☐	
Star Jumps	40	☐	40	☐	40	☐	40	☐	40	☐	40	☐	
Squat Thrusts	20	☐	20	☐	20	☐	20	☐	20	☐	20	☐	
Step Ups	40	☐	40	☐	40	☐	40	☐	40	☐	40	☐	
Run / Jog	3 mins	☐	3 mins	☐	3 mins	☐	3 mins	☐	3 mins	☐	3 mins	☐	

Exercise Resolution
By Andrew Banks

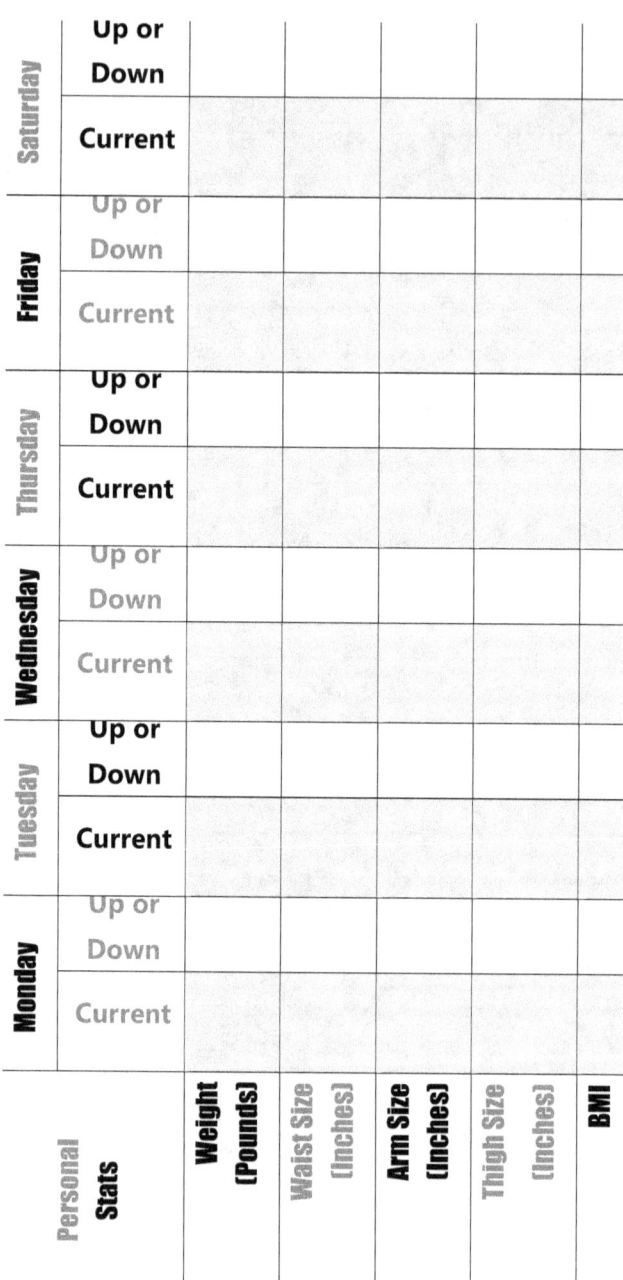

Progress Chart—Week 17

Personal Stats	Monday Current	Monday Up or Down	Tuesday Current	Tuesday Up or Down	Wednesday Current	Wednesday Up or Down	Thursday Current	Thursday Up or Down	Friday Current	Friday Up or Down	Saturday Current	Saturday Up or Down
Weight (Pounds)												
Waist Size (Inches)												
Arm Size (Inches)												
Thigh Size (Inches)												
BMI												

BMI Calculation

$$BMI = \frac{(\text{Weight in pounds} \times 703)}{(\text{Height in Inches} \times \text{Height in Inches})}$$

If you are unsure about working out any of these statistics then please refer to the main guide book which will explain these to you in more detail and help you to understand it better. Remember, you are doing well, keep it up.

Exercise Resolution
By Andrew Banks

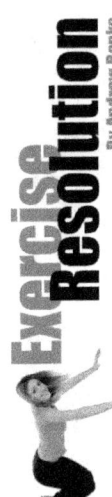

Progress Chart—Week 19

Exercise	Monday Required	Monday Complete?	Tuesday Required	Tuesday Complete?	Wednesday Required	Wednesday Complete?	Thursday Required	Thursday Complete?	Friday Required	Friday Complete?	Saturday Required	Saturday Complete?	Total
Push Ups	20	☐	20	☐	20	☐	20	☐	20	☐	20	☐	
Sit Ups	20	☐	20	☐	20	☐	20	☐	20	☐	20	☐	
Star Jumps	40	☐	40	☐	40	☐	40	☐	40	☐	40	☐	
Squat Thrusts	20	☐	20	☐	20	☐	20	☐	20	☐	20	☐	
Step Ups	40	☐	40	☐	40	☐	40	☐	40	☐	40	☐	
Run / Jog	3 mins	☐	3 mins	☐	3 mins	☐	3 mins	☐	3 mins	☐	3 mins	☐	

Exercise Resolution
By Andrew Banks

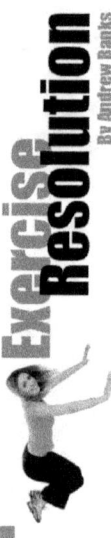

Progress Chart—Week 19

Personal Stats	Monday		Tuesday		Wednesday		Thursday		Friday		Saturday	
	Current	Up or Down	Current	Up or Down	Current	Up or Down	Current	Up or Down	Current	Up or Down	Current	Up or Down
Weight (Pounds)												
Waist Size (Inches)												
Arm Size (Inches)												
Thigh Size (Inches)												
BMI												

BMI Calculation

$$BMI = \frac{(\text{Weight in pounds} \times 703)}{(\text{Height in Inches} \times \text{Height in Inches})}$$

If you are unsure about working out any of these statistics then please refer to the main guide book which will explain these to you in more detail and help you to understand it better. Remember, you are doing well, keep it up.

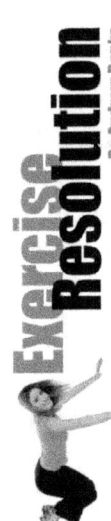

Exercise Resolution
By Andrew Banks

Progress Chart—Week 19

Exercise	Monday Required	Monday Complete?	Tuesday Required	Tuesday Complete?	Wednesday Required	Wednesday Complete?	Thursday Required	Thursday Complete?	Friday Required	Friday Complete?	Saturday Required	Saturday Complete?	Total
Push Ups 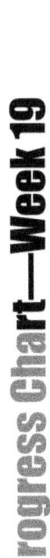	20	☐	20	☐	20	☐	20	☐	20	☐	20	☐	
Sit Ups	20	☐	20	☐	20	☐	20	☐	20	☐	20	☐	
Star Jumps	40	☐	40	☐	40	☐	40	☐	40	☐	40	☐	
Squat Thrusts	20	☐	20	☐	20	☐	20	☐	20	☐	20	☐	
Step Ups	40	☐	40	☐	40	☐	40	☐	40	☐	40	☐	
Run / Jog	3 mins	☐	3 mins	☐	3 mins	☐	3 mins	☐	3 mins	☐	3 mins	☐	

Exercise Resolution
By Andrew Banks

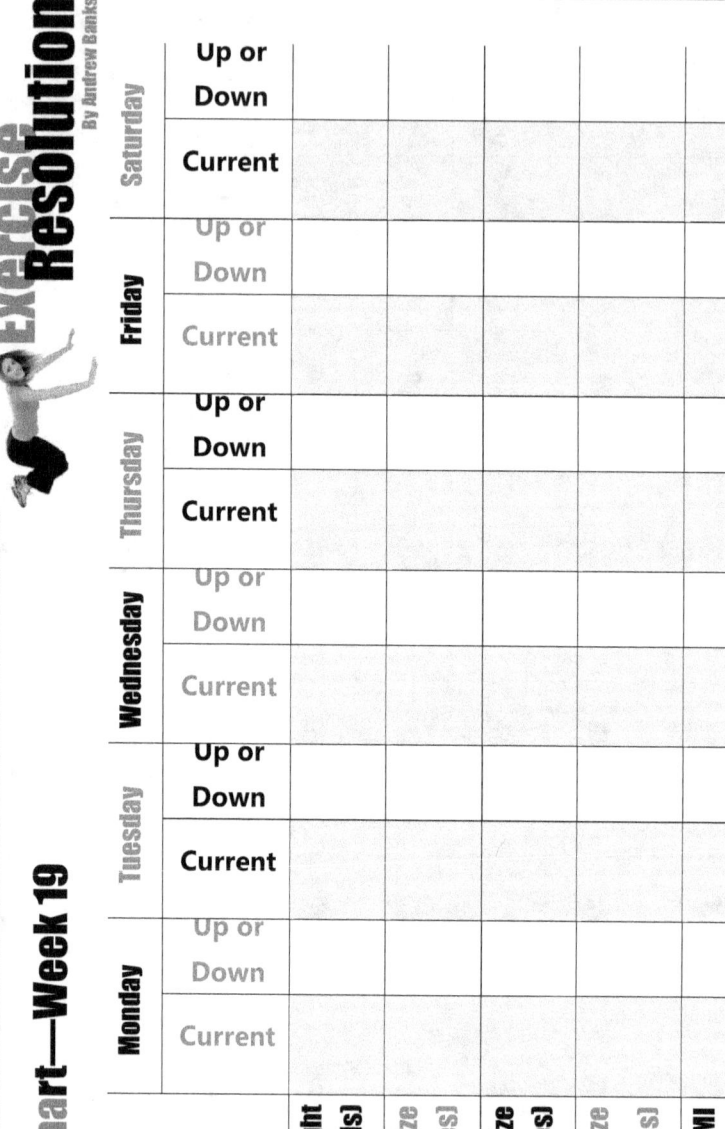

Progress Chart—Week 19

Personal Stats	Monday		Tuesday		Wednesday		Thursday		Friday		Saturday	
	Current	Up or Down	Current	Up or Down	Current	Up or Down	Current	Up or Down	Current	Up or Down	Current	Up or Down
Weight (Pounds)												
Waist Size (Inches)												
Arm Size (Inches)												
Thigh Size (Inches)												
BMI												

BMI Calculation

$$BMI = \frac{(\text{Weight in pounds} \times 703)}{(\text{Height in Inches} \times \text{Height in Inches})}$$

If you are unsure about working out any of these statistics then please refer to the main guide book which will explain these to you in more detail and help you to understand it better. Remember, you are doing well, keep it up.

Exercise Resolution
By Andrew Banks

Progress Chart—Week 2

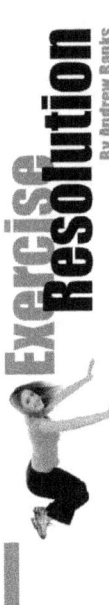

Exercise	Monday Required	Monday Complete?	Tuesday Required	Tuesday Complete?	Wednesday Required	Wednesday Complete?	Thursday Required	Thursday Complete?	Friday Required	Friday Complete?	Saturday Required	Saturday Complete?	Total
Push Ups	6	☐	6	☐	7	☐	7	☐	9	☐	9	☐	
Sit Ups	6	☐	6	☐	7	☐	7	☐	9	☐	9	☐	
Star Jumps	10	☐	10	☐	15	☐	15	☐	20	☐	20	☐	
Squat Thrusts	6	☐	6	☐	7	☐	7	☐	7	☐	7	☐	
Step Ups	20	☐	20	☐	24	☐	24	☐	26	☐	26	☐	
Run / Jog	-	☐	-	☐	-	☐	-	☐	-	☐	-	☐	

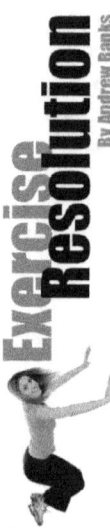

Exercise Resolution
By Andrew Banks

Progress Chart—Week 2

Personal Stats	Monday		Tuesday		Wednesday		Thursday		Friday		Saturday	
	Current	Up or Down	Current	Up or Down	Current	Up or Down	Current	Up or Down	Current	Up or Down	Current	Up or Down
Weight (Pounds)												
Waist Size (Inches)												
Arm Size (Inches)												
Thigh Size (Inches)												
BMI												

BMI Calculation

$$BMI = \frac{(\text{Weight in pounds} \times 703)}{(\text{Height in Inches} \times \text{Height in Inches})}$$

If you are unsure about working out any of these statistics then please refer to the main guide book which will explain these to you in more detail and help you to understand it better. Remember, you are doing well, keep it up.

Exercise Resolution
By Andrew Banks

Progress Chart—Week 20

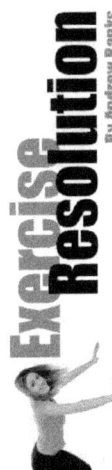

Exercise	Monday Required	Monday Complete?	Tuesday Required	Tuesday Complete?	Wednesday Required	Wednesday Complete?	Thursday Required	Thursday Complete?	Friday Required	Friday Complete?	Saturday Required	Saturday Complete?	Total
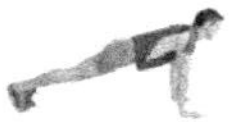 Push Ups	20	☐	20	☐	22	☐	22	☐	24	☐	24	☐	
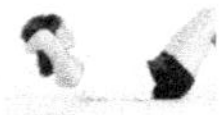 Sit Ups	20	☐	20	☐	22	☐	22	☐	24	☐	24	☐	
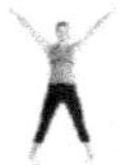 Star Jumps	42	☐	42	☐	44	☐	44	☐	46	☐	46	☐	
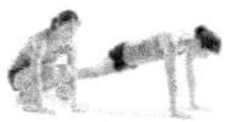 Squat Thrusts	20	☐	20	☐	22	☐	22	☐	24	☐	24	☐	
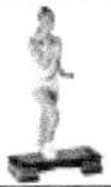 Step Ups	42	☐	42	☐	44	☐	44	☐	46	☐	46	☐	
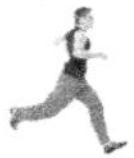 Run / Jog	3 mins	☐	3 mins	☐	3 mins	☐	3 mins	☐	3 mins	☐	4 mins	☐	

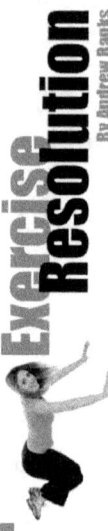

Exercise Resolution
By Andrew Banks

Progress Chart—Week 20

Personal Stats	Monday		Tuesday		Wednesday		Thursday		Friday		Saturday	
	Current	Up or Down	Current	Up or Down	Current	Up or Down	Current	Up or Down	Current	Up or Down	Current	Up or Down
Weight (Pounds)												
Waist Size (Inches)												
Arm Size (Inches)												
Thigh Size (Inches)												
BMI												

BMI Calculation

$$BMI = \frac{(\text{Weight in pounds} \times 703\,)}{(\text{Height in Inches} \times \text{Height in Inches})}$$

If you are unsure about working out any of these statistics then please refer to the main guide book which will explain these to you in more detail and help you to understand it better. Remember, you are doing well, keep it up.

Exercise Resolution
By Andrew Banks

Progress Chart—Week 21

Exercise	Monday Required	Monday Complete?	Tuesday Required	Tuesday Complete?	Wednesday Required	Wednesday Complete?	Thursday Required	Thursday Complete?	Friday Required	Friday Complete?	Saturday Required	Saturday Complete?	Total
Push Ups	22	☐	22	☐	24	☐	24	☐	26	☐	26	☐	
Sit Ups	22	☐	22	☐	24	☐	24	☐	26	☐	26	☐	
Star Jumps	44	☐	44	☐	46	☐	46	☐	48	☐	48	☐	
Squat Thrusts	22	☐	22	☐	24	☐	24	☐	26	☐	26	☐	
Step Ups	44	☐	44	☐	46	☐	46	☐	48	☐	48	☐	
Run / Jog	3 mins	☐	3 mins	☐	3 mins	☐	3 mins	☐	4 mins	☐	4 mins	☐	

Exercise Resolution
By Andrew Banks

Progress Chart—Week 21

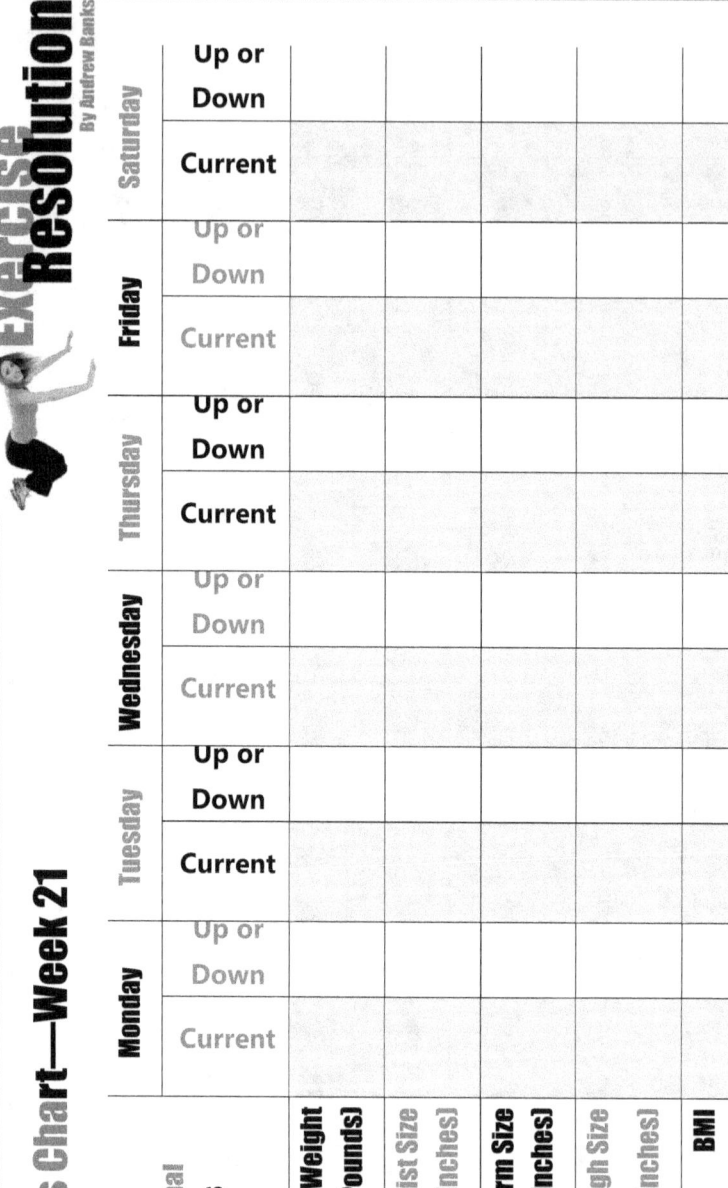

Personal Stats	Monday Current	Monday Up or Down	Tuesday Current	Tuesday Up or Down	Wednesday Current	Wednesday Up or Down	Thursday Current	Thursday Up or Down	Friday Current	Friday Up or Down	Saturday Current	Saturday Up or Down
Weight (Pounds)												
Waist Size (Inches)												
Arm Size (Inches)												
Thigh Size (Inches)												
BMI												

BMI Calculation

$$BMI = \frac{(\text{Weight in pounds} \times 703)}{(\text{Height in Inches} \times \text{Height in Inches})}$$

If you are unsure about working out any of these statistics then please refer to the main guide book which will explain these to you in more detail and help you to understand it better. Remember, you are doing well, keep it up.

Exercise Resolution
By Andrew Banks

Progress Chart—Week 22

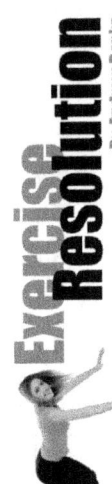

Exercise	Monday Required	Monday Complete?	Tuesday Required	Tuesday Complete?	Wednesday Required	Wednesday Complete?	Thursday Required	Thursday Complete?	Friday Required	Friday Complete?	Saturday Required	Saturday Complete?	Total
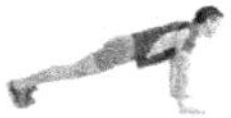 Push Ups	24	☐	24	☐	26	☐	26	☐	28	☐	28	☐	
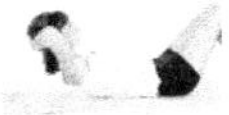 Sit Ups	24	☐	24	☐	26	☐	26	☐	28	☐	28	☐	
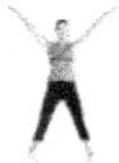 Star Jumps	46	☐	46	☐	48	☐	48	☐	50	☐	50	☐	
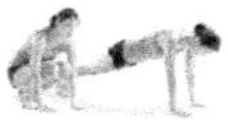 Squat Thrusts	24	☐	24	☐	26	☐	26	☐	28	☐	28	☐	
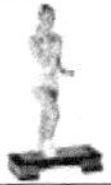 Step Ups	46	☐	46	☐	48	☐	48	☐	50	☐	50	☐	
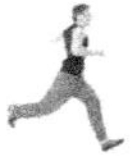 Run / Jog	3 mins	☐	3 mins	☐	3 mins	☐	4 mins	☐	4 mins	☐	4 mins	☐	

Exercise Resolution
By Andrew Banks

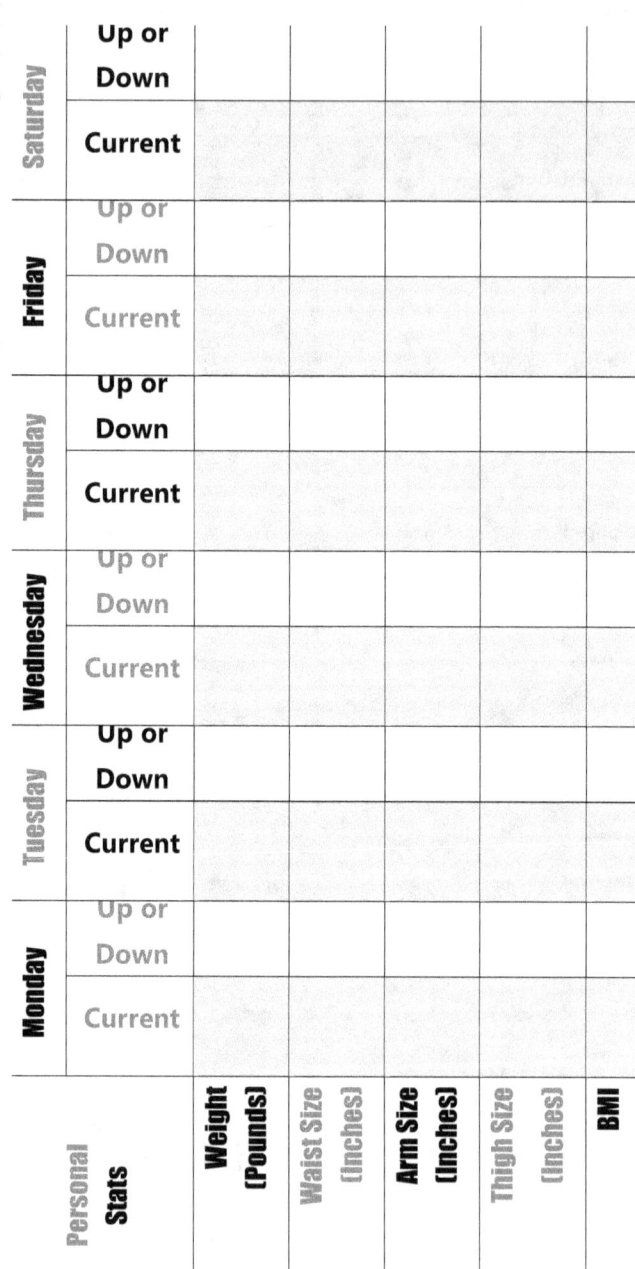

Progress Chart—Week 22

Personal Stats	Monday		Tuesday		Wednesday		Thursday		Friday		Saturday	
	Current	Up or Down	Current	Up or Down	Current	Up or Down	Current	Up or Down	Current	Up or Down	Current	Up or Down
Weight (Pounds)												
Waist Size (Inches)												
Arm Size (Inches)												
Thigh Size (Inches)												
BMI												

BMI Calculation

$$BMI = \frac{(\text{Weight in pounds} \times 703)}{(\text{Height in Inches} \times \text{Height in Inches})}$$

If you are unsure about working out any of these statistics then please refer to the main guide book which will explain these to you in more detail and help you to understand it better. Remember, you are doing well, keep it up.

Exercise Resolution
By Andrew Banks

Progress Chart—Week 23

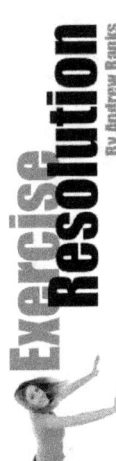

Exercise	Monday Required	Monday Complete?	Tuesday Required	Tuesday Complete?	Wednesday Required	Wednesday Complete?	Thursday Required	Thursday Complete?	Friday Required	Friday Complete?	Saturday Required	Saturday Complete?	Total
Push Ups	26	☐	26	☐	28	☐	28	☐	30	☐	30	☐	
Sit Ups	26	☐	26	☐	28	☐	28	☐	30	☐	30	☐	
Star Jumps	48	☐	48	☐	50	☐	50	☐	50	☐	50	☐	
Squat Thrusts	26	☐	26	☐	28	☐	28	☐	30	☐	30	☐	
Step Ups	48	☐	48	☐	50	☐	50	☐	50	☐	50	☐	
Run / Jog	3 mins	☐	3 mins	☐	4 mins	☐	4 mins	☐	4 mins	☐	4 mins	☐	

Exercise Resolution
By Andrew Banks

Progress Chart—Week 23

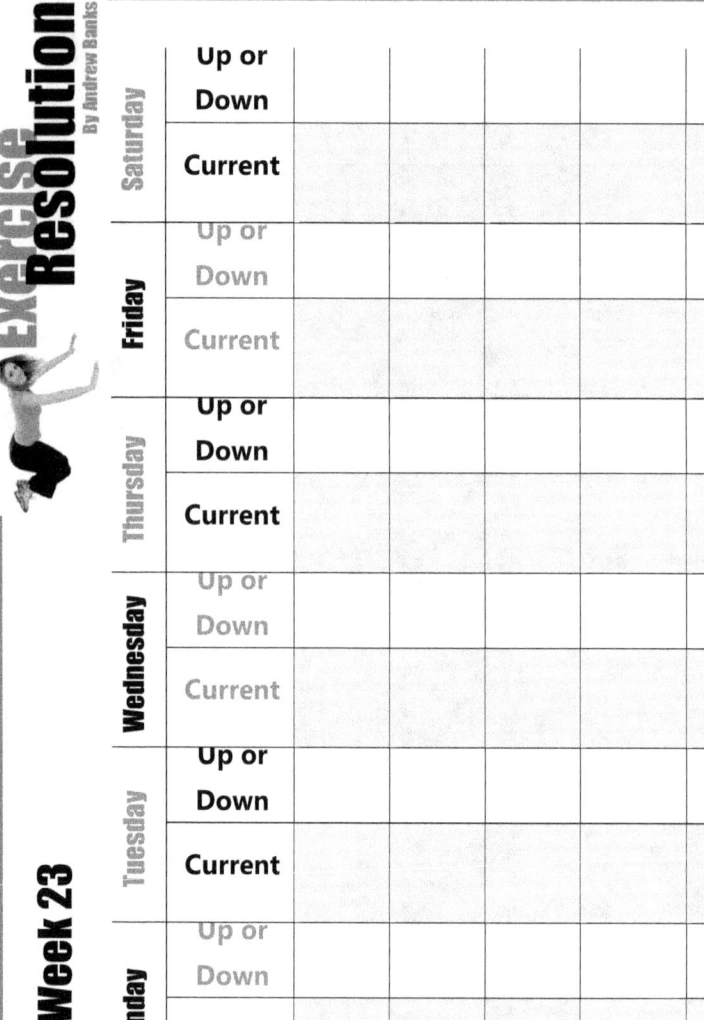

Personal Stats	Monday		Tuesday		Wednesday		Thursday		Friday		Saturday	
	Current	Up or Down	Current	Up or Down	Current	Up or Down	Current	Up or Down	Current	Up or Down	Current	Up or Down
Weight (Pounds)												
Waist Size (Inches)												
Arm Size (Inches)												
Thigh Size (Inches)												
BMI												

BMI Calculation

$$BMI = \frac{(\text{Weight in pounds} \times 703)}{(\text{Height in Inches} \times \text{Height in Inches})}$$

If you are unsure about working out any of these statistics then please refer to the main guide book which will explain these to you in more detail and help you to understand it better. Remember, you are doing well, keep it up.

Exercise Resolution
By Andrew Banks

Progress Chart—Week 24

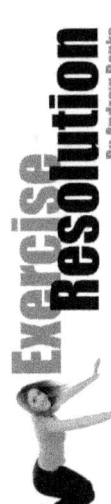

Exercise	Monday Required	Monday Complete?	Tuesday Required	Tuesday Complete?	Wednesday Required	Wednesday Complete?	Thursday Required	Thursday Complete?	Friday Required	Friday Complete?	Saturday Required	Saturday Complete?	Total
Push Ups	28	☐	28	☐	30	☐	30	☐	30	☐	30	☐	
Sit Ups	28	☐	28	☐	30	☐	30	☐	30	☐	30	☐	
Star Jumps	50	☐	50	☐	50	☐	50	☐	50	☐	50	☐	
Squat Thrusts	28	☐	28	☐	30	☐	30	☐	30	☐	30	☐	
Step Ups	50	☐	50	☐	50	☐	50	☐	50	☐	50	☐	
Run / Jog	3 mins	☐	3 mins	☐	4 mins	☐	4 mins	☐	4 mins	☐	4 mins	☐	

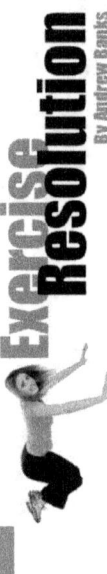

Exercise Resolution
By Andrew Banks

Progress Chart—Week 24

Personal Stats	Monday Current	Monday Up or Down	Tuesday Current	Tuesday Up or Down	Wednesday Current	Wednesday Up or Down	Thursday Current	Thursday Up or Down	Friday Current	Friday Up or Down	Saturday Current	Saturday Up or Down
Weight (Pounds)												
Waist Size (Inches)												
Arm Size (Inches)												
Thigh Size (Inches)												
BMI												

BMI Calculation

$$BMI = \frac{(\text{Weight in pounds} \times 703)}{(\text{Height in Inches} \times \text{Height in Inches})}$$

If you are unsure about working out any of these statistics then please refer to the main guide book which will explain these to you in more detail and help you to understand it better. Remember, you are doing well, keep it up.

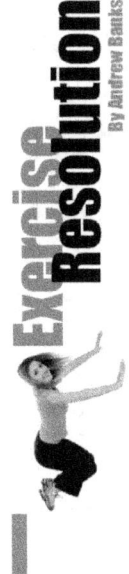

Exercise ResoIution
By Andrew Banks

Progress Chart—Week 25

Exercise	Monday Required	Monday Complete?	Tuesday Required	Tuesday Complete?	Wednesday Required	Wednesday Complete?	Thursday Required	Thursday Complete?	Friday Required	Friday Complete?	Saturday Required	Saturday Complete?	Total
Push Ups	30	☐	30	☐	30	☐	30	☐	30	☐	30	☐	
Sit Ups	30	☐	30	☐	30	☐	30	☐	30	☐	30	☐	
Star Jumps	50	☐	50	☐	50	☐	50	☐	50	☐	50	☐	
Squat Thrusts	30	☐	30	☐	30	☐	30	☐	30	☐	30	☐	
Step Ups	50	☐	50	☐	50	☐	50	☐	50	☐	50	☐	
Run / Jog	3 mins	☐	4 mins	☐	4 mins	☐	4 mins	☐	4 mins	☐	4 mins	☐	

Exercise Resolution
By Andrew Banks

Progress Chart—Week 25

Personal Stats	Monday		Tuesday		Wednesday		Thursday		Friday		Saturday	
	Current	Up or Down	Current	Up or Down	Current	Up or Down	Current	Up or Down	Current	Up or Down	Current	Up or Down
Weight (Pounds)												
Waist Size (Inches)												
Arm Size (Inches)												
Thigh Size (Inches)												
BMI												

If you are unsure about working out any of these statistics then please refer to the main guide book which will explain these to you in more detail and help you to understand it better. Remember, you are doing well, keep it up.

BMI Calculation

$$BMI = \frac{(Weight\ in\ pounds \times 703)}{(Height\ in\ Inches \times Height\ in\ Inches)}$$

Exercise Resolution
By Andrew Banks

Progress Chart—Week 26

Exercise	Monday Required	Monday Complete?	Tuesday Required	Tuesday Complete?	Wednesday Required	Wednesday Complete?	Thursday Required	Thursday Complete?	Friday Required	Friday Complete?	Saturday Required	Saturday Complete?	Total
Push Ups	30	☐	30	☐	30	☐	30	☐	30	☐	30	☐	
Sit Ups	30	☐	30	☐	30	☐	30	☐	30	☐	30	☐	
Star Jumps	50	☐	50	☐	50	☐	50	☐	50	☐	50	☐	
Squat Thrusts	30	☐	30	☐	30	☐	30	☐	30	☐	30	☐	
Step Ups	50	☐	50	☐	50	☐	50	☐	50	☐	50	☐	
Run / Jog	4 mins	☐	4 mins	☐	4 mins	☐	4 mins	☐	4 mins	☐	4 mins	☐	

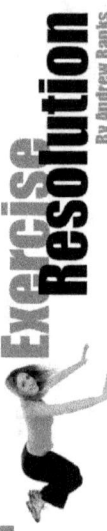

Exercise Resolution
By Andrew Banks

Progress Chart—Week 26

Personal Stats	Monday Current	Monday Up or Down	Tuesday Current	Tuesday Up or Down	Wednesday Current	Wednesday Up or Down	Thursday Current	Thursday Up or Down	Friday Current	Friday Up or Down	Saturday Current	Saturday Up or Down
Weight (Pounds)												
Waist Size (Inches)												
Arm Size (Inches)												
Thigh Size (Inches)												
BMI												

BMI Calculation

$$BMI = \frac{(\text{Weight in pounds} \times 703)}{(\text{Height in Inches} \times \text{Height in Inches})}$$

If you are unsure about working out any of these statistics then please refer to the main guide book which will explain these to you in more detail and help you to understand it better. Remember, you are doing well, keep it up.

Exercise Resolution
By Andrew Banks

Progress Chart—Week 27

Exercise	Monday Required	Monday Complete?	Tuesday Required	Tuesday Complete?	Wednesday Required	Wednesday Complete?	Thursday Required	Thursday Complete?	Friday Required	Friday Complete?	Saturday Required	Saturday Complete?	Total
Push Ups	30	☐	30	☐	30	☐	30	☐	30	☐	30	☐	
Sit Ups	30	☐	30	☐	30	☐	30	☐	30	☐	30	☐	
Star Jumps	50	☐	50	☐	50	☐	50	☐	50	☐	50	☐	
Squat Thrusts	30	☐	30	☐	30	☐	30	☐	30	☐	30	☐	
Step Ups	50	☐	50	☐	50	☐	50	☐	50	☐	50	☐	
Run / Jog	4 mins	☐	4 mins	☐	4 mins	☐	4 mins	☐	4 mins	☐	4 mins	☐	

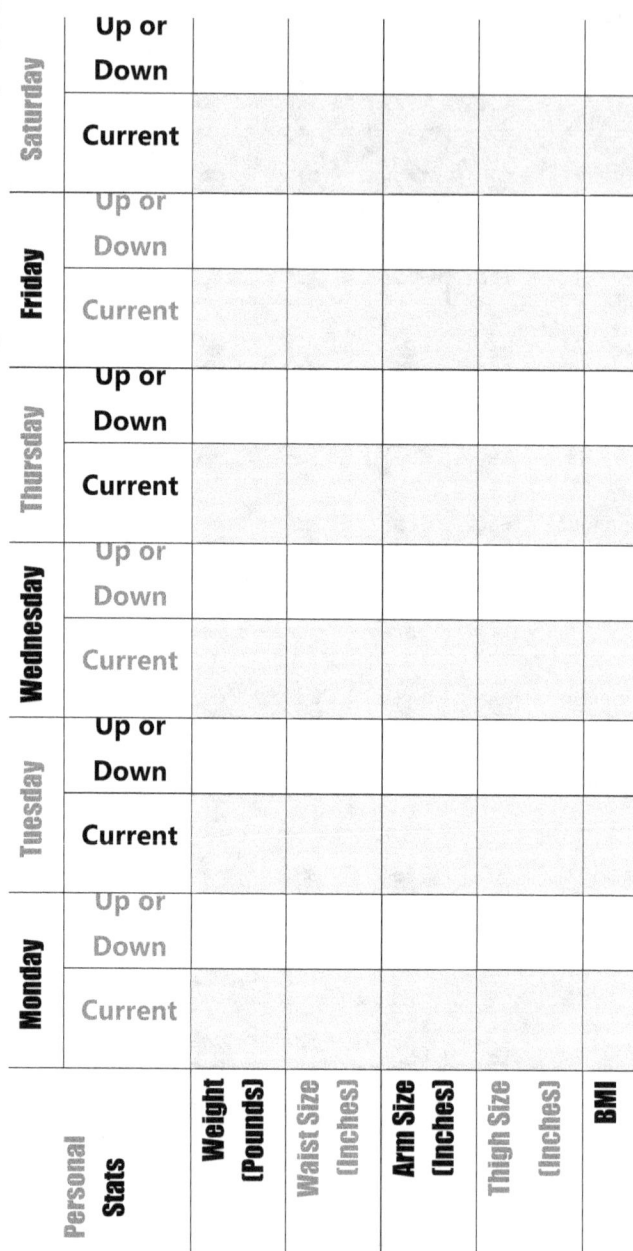

Exercise Resolution
By Andrew Banks

Progress Chart—Week 27

Personal Stats	Monday Current	Monday Up or Down	Tuesday Current	Tuesday Up or Down	Wednesday Current	Wednesday Up or Down	Thursday Current	Thursday Up or Down	Friday Current	Friday Up or Down	Saturday Current	Saturday Up or Down
Weight (Pounds)												
Waist Size (Inches)												
Arm Size (Inches)												
Thigh Size (Inches)												
BMI												

BMI Calculation

$$BMI = \frac{(\text{Weight in pounds} \times 703)}{(\text{Height in Inches} \times \text{Height in Inches})}$$

If you are unsure about working out any of these statistics then please refer to the main guide book which will explain these to you in more detail and help you to understand it better. Remember, you are doing well, keep it up.

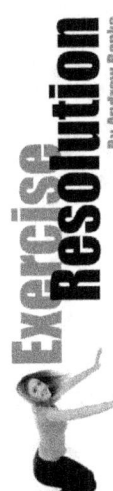

Exercise Resolution
By Andrew Banks

Progress Chart—Week 28

Exercise	Monday Required	Monday Complete?	Tuesday Required	Tuesday Complete?	Wednesday Required	Wednesday Complete?	Thursday Required	Thursday Complete?	Friday Required	Friday Complete?	Saturday Required	Saturday Complete?	Total
Push Ups	30	☐	30	☐	30	☐	30	☐	30	☐	30	☐	
Sit Ups	30	☐	30	☐	30	☐	30	☐	30	☐	30	☐	
Star Jumps	50	☐	50	☐	50	☐	50	☐	50	☐	50	☐	
Squat Thrusts	30	☐	30	☐	30	☐	30	☐	30	☐	30	☐	
Step Ups	50	☐	50	☐	50	☐	50	☐	50	☐	50	☐	
Run / Jog	4 mins	☐	4 mins	☐	4 mins	☐	4 mins	☐	4 mins	☐	4 mins	☐	

Exercise Resolution
By Andrew Banks

Progress Chart—Week 28

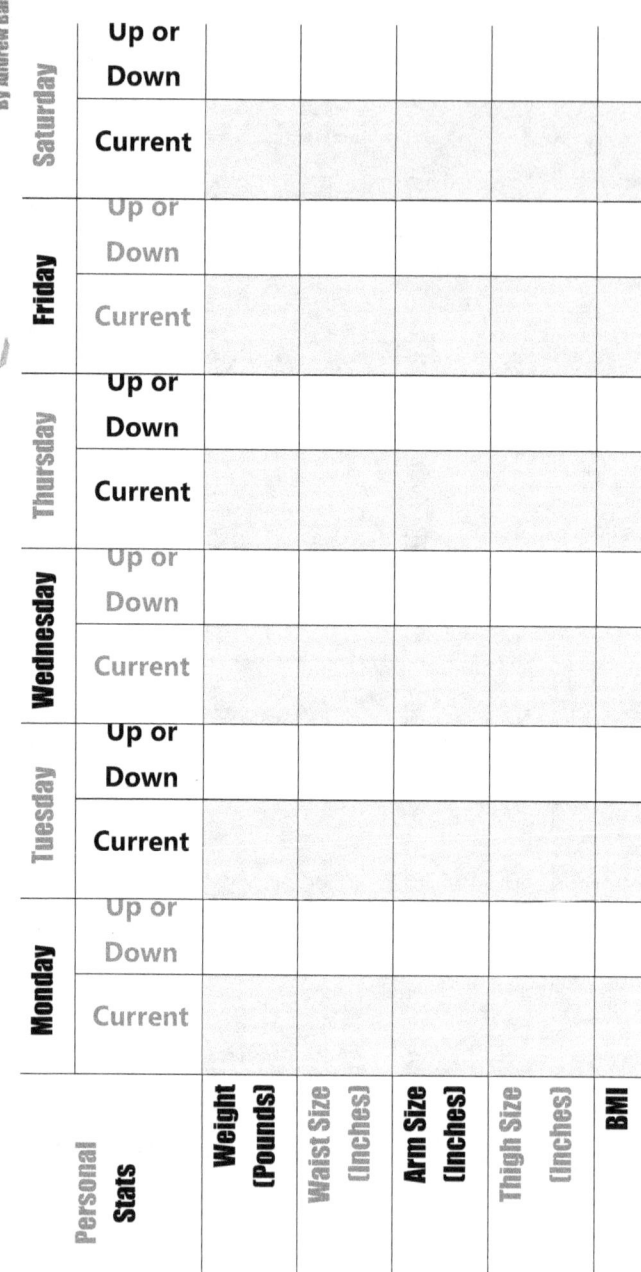

Personal Stats	Monday		Tuesday		Wednesday		Thursday		Friday		Saturday	
	Current	Up or Down	Current	Up or Down	Current	Up or Down	Current	Up or Down	Current	Up or Down	Current	Up or Down
Weight (Pounds)												
Waist Size (Inches)												
Arm Size (Inches)												
Thigh Size (Inches)												
BMI												

BMI Calculation

$$BMI = \frac{(\text{Weight in pounds} \times 703)}{(\text{Height in Inches} \times \text{Height in Inches})}$$

If you are unsure about working out any of these statistics then please refer to the main guide book which will explain these to you in more detail and help you to understand it better. Remember, you are doing well, keep it up.

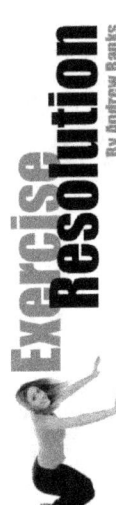

Exercise Resolution
By Andrew Banks

Progress Chart—Week 29

Exercise	Monday Required	Monday Complete?	Tuesday Required	Tuesday Complete?	Wednesday Required	Wednesday Complete?	Thursday Required	Thursday Complete?	Friday Required	Friday Complete?	Saturday Required	Saturday Complete?	Total
Push Ups	30	☐	30	☐	32	☐	32	☐	34	☐	34	☐	
Sit Ups	30	☐	30	☐	32	☐	32	☐	34	☐	34	☐	
Star Jumps	52	☐	52	☐	54	☐	54	☐	56	☐	56	☐	
Squat Thrusts	30	☐	30	☐	32	☐	32	☐	34	☐	34	☐	
Step Ups	52	☐	52	☐	54	☐	54	☐	56	☐	56	☐	
Run / Jog	4 mins	☐	4 mins	☐	4 mins	☐	4 mins	☐	4 mins	☐	5 mins	☐	

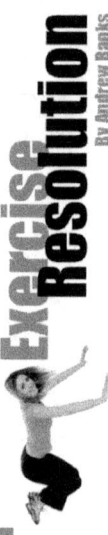

Exercise Resolution
By Andrew Banks

Progress Chart—Week 29

Personal Stats	Monday		Tuesday		Wednesday		Thursday		Friday		Saturday	
	Current	Up or Down	Current	Up or Down	Current	Up or Down	Current	Up or Down	Current	Up or Down	Current	Up or Down
Weight (Pounds)												
Waist Size (Inches)												
Arm Size (Inches)												
Thigh Size (Inches)												
BMI												

BMI Calculation

$$BMI = \frac{(\text{Weight in pounds} \times 703)}{(\text{Height in Inches} \times \text{Height in Inches})}$$

If you are unsure about working out any of these statistics then please refer to the main guide book which will explain these to you in more detail and help you to understand it better. Remember, you are doing well, keep it up.

Exercise Resolution

By Andrew Banks

Progress Chart—Week 3

Exercise	Monday Required	Monday Complete?	Tuesday Required	Tuesday Complete?	Wednesday Required	Wednesday Complete?	Thursday Required	Thursday Complete?	Friday Required	Friday Complete?	Saturday Required	Saturday Complete?	Total
Push Ups	7	☐	7	☐	8	☐	8	☐	10	☐	10	☐	
Sit Ups	7	☐	7	☐	8	☐	8	☐	10	☐	10	☐	
Star Jumps	15	☐	15	☐	20	☐	20	☐	25	☐	25	☐	
Squat Thrusts	7	☐	7	☐	8	☐	8	☐	10	☐	10	☐	
Step Ups	24	☐	24	☐	26	☐	26	☐	30	☐	30	☐	
Run / Jog	-	☐	-	☐	-	☐	-	☐	-	☐	-	☐	

Exercise Resolution
By Andrew Banks

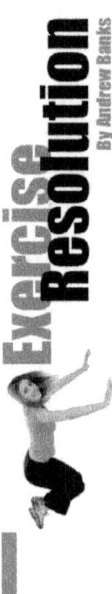

Progress Chart—Week 3

Personal Stats	Monday		Tuesday		Wednesday		Thursday		Friday		Saturday	
	Current	Up or Down	Current	Up or Down	Current	Up or Down	Current	Up or Down	Current	Up or Down	Current	Up or Down
Weight (Pounds)												
Waist Size (Inches)												
Arm Size (Inches)												
Thigh Size (Inches)												
BMI												

BMI Calculation

$$BMI = \frac{(Weight\ in\ pounds \times 703)}{(Height\ in\ Inches \times Height\ in\ Inches)}$$

If you are unsure about working out any of these statistics then please refer to the main guide book which will explain these to you in more detail and help you to understand it better. Remember, you are doing well, keep it up.

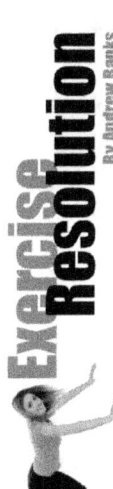

Exercise Resolution
By Andrew Banks

Progress Chart—Week 30

Exercise	Monday Required	Monday Complete?	Tuesday Required	Tuesday Complete?	Wednesday Required	Wednesday Complete?	Thursday Required	Thursday Complete?	Friday Required	Friday Complete?	Saturday Required	Saturday Complete?	Total
Push Ups	32	☐	32	☐	34	☐	34	☐	36	☐	36	☐	
Sit Ups	32	☐	32	☐	34	☐	34	☐	36	☐	36	☐	
Star Jumps	54	☐	54	☐	56	☐	56	☐	58	☐	58	☐	
Squat Thrusts	32	☐	32	☐	34	☐	34	☐	36	☐	36	☐	
Step Ups	54	☐	54	☐	56	☐	56	☐	58	☐	58	☐	
Run / Jog	4 mins	☐	4 mins	☐	4 mins	☐	4 mins	☐	5 mins	☐	5 mins	☐	

Exercise Resolution
By Andrew Banks

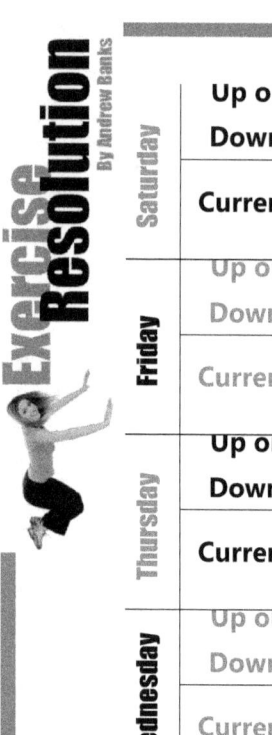

Progress Chart—Week 30

Personal Stats	Monday		Tuesday		Wednesday		Thursday		Friday		Saturday	
	Current	Up or Down	Current	Up or Down	Current	Up or Down	Current	Up or Down	Current	Up or Down	Current	Up or Down
Weight (Pounds)												
Waist Size (Inches)												
Arm Size (Inches)												
Thigh Size (Inches)												
BMI												

BMI Calculation

$$BMI = \frac{(\text{Weight in pounds} \times 703)}{(\text{Height in Inches} \times \text{Height in Inches})}$$

If you are unsure about working out any of these statistics then please refer to the main guide book which will explain these to you in more detail and help you to understand it better. Remember, you are doing well, keep it up.

Exercise Resolution
By Andrew Banks

Progress Chart—Week 4

Exercise	Monday Required	Monday Complete?	Tuesday Required	Tuesday Complete?	Wednesday Required	Wednesday Complete?	Thursday Required	Thursday Complete?	Friday Required	Friday Complete?	Saturday Required	Saturday Complete?	Total
Push Ups	8	☐	8	☐	10	☐	10	☐	10	☐	10	☐	
Sit Ups	8	☐	8	☐	10	☐	10	☐	10	☐	10	☐	
Star Jumps	20	☐	20	☐	25	☐	25	☐	30	☐	30	☐	
Squat Thrusts	8	☐	8	☐	10	☐	10	☐	10	☐	10	☐	
Step Ups	26	☐	26	☐	30	☐	30	☐	30	☐	30	☐	
Run / Jog	'	☐	'	☐	'	☐	'	☐	'	☐	'	☐	

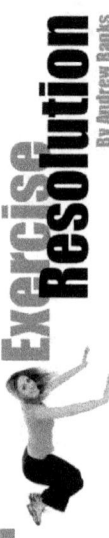

Exercise Resolution
By Andrew Banks

Progress Chart—Week 4

Personal Stats	Monday		Tuesday		Wednesday		Thursday		Friday		Saturday	
	Current	Up or Down	Current	Up or Down	Current	Up or Down	Current	Up or Down	Current	Up or Down	Current	Up or Down
Weight (Pounds)												
Waist Size (Inches)												
Arm Size (Inches)												
Thigh Size (Inches)												
BMI												

BMI Calculation

$$BMI = \frac{(\text{Weight in pounds} \times 703)}{(\text{Height in Inches} \times \text{Height in Inches})}$$

If you are unsure about working out any of these statistics then please refer to the main guide book which will explain these to you in more detail and help you to understand it better. Remember, you are doing well, keep it up.

Exercise Resolution
By Andrew Banks

Progress Chart—Week 5

Exercise	Monday Required	Monday Complete?	Tuesday Required	Tuesday Complete?	Wednesday Required	Wednesday Complete?	Thursday Required	Thursday Complete?	Friday Required	Friday Complete?	Saturday Required	Saturday Complete?	Total
Push Ups	7	☐	7	☐	8	☐	8	☐	10	☐	10	☐	
Sit Ups	7	☐	7	☐	8	☐	8	☐	10	☐	10	☐	
Star Jumps	15	☐	15	☐	20	☐	20	☐	25	☐	25	☐	
Squat Thrusts	7	☐	7	☐	8	☐	8	☐	10	☐	10	☐	
Step Ups	24	☐	24	☐	26	☐	26	☐	30	☐	30	☐	
Run / Jog	2 mins	☐	2 mins	☐	2 mins	☐	2 mins	☐	2 mins	☐	2 mins	☐	

Exercise Resolution
By Andrew Banks

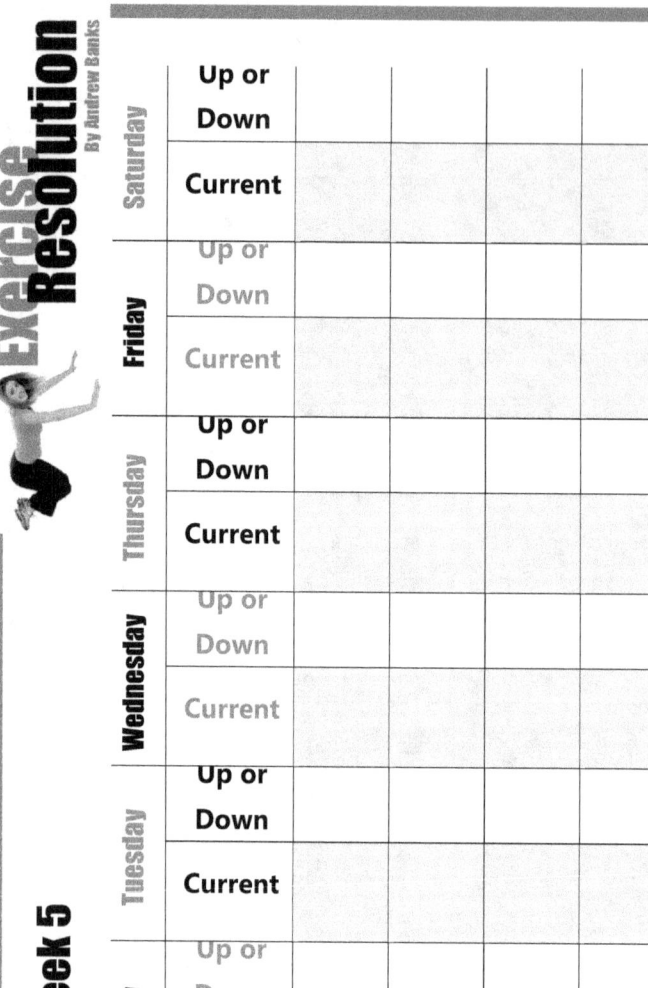

Progress Chart—Week 5

Personal Stats	Monday		Tuesday		Wednesday		Thursday		Friday		Saturday	
	Current	Up or Down	Current	Up or Down	Current	Up or Down	Current	Up or Down	Current	Up or Down	Current	Up or Down
Weight (Pounds)												
Waist Size (Inches)												
Arm Size (Inches)												
Thigh Size (Inches)												
BMI												

BMI Calculation

$$BMI = \frac{(\text{Weight in pounds} \times 703)}{(\text{Height in Inches} \times \text{Height in Inches})}$$

If you are unsure about working out any of these statistics then please refer to the main guide book which will explain these to you in more detail and help you to understand it better. Remember, you are doing well, keep it up.

Exercise Resolution
By Andrew Banks

Progress Chart—Week 6

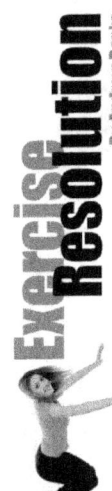

Exercise	Monday Required	Monday Complete?	Tuesday Required	Tuesday Complete?	Wednesday Required	Wednesday Complete?	Thursday Required	Thursday Complete?	Friday Required	Friday Complete?	Saturday Required	Saturday Complete?	Total
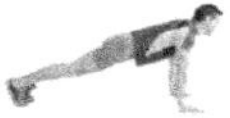 Push Ups	8	☐	8	☐	10	☐	10	☐	10	☐	10	☐	
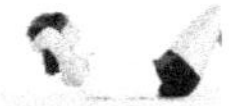 Sit Ups	8	☐	8	☐	10	☐	10	☐	10	☐	10	☐	
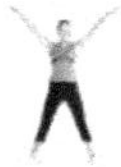 Star Jumps	20	☐	20	☐	25	☐	25	☐	30	☐	30	☐	
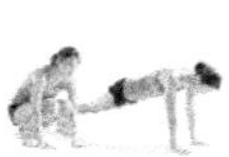 Squat Thrusts	8	☐	8	☐	10	☐	10	☐	10	☐	10	☐	
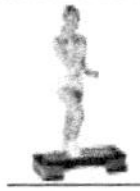 Step Ups	26	☐	26	☐	30	☐	30	☐	30	☐	30	☐	
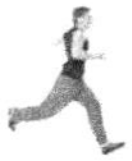 Run / Jog	2 mins	☐	2 mins	☐	2 mins	☐	2 mins	☐	2 mins	☐	2 mins	☐	

Exercise Resolution
By Andrew Banks

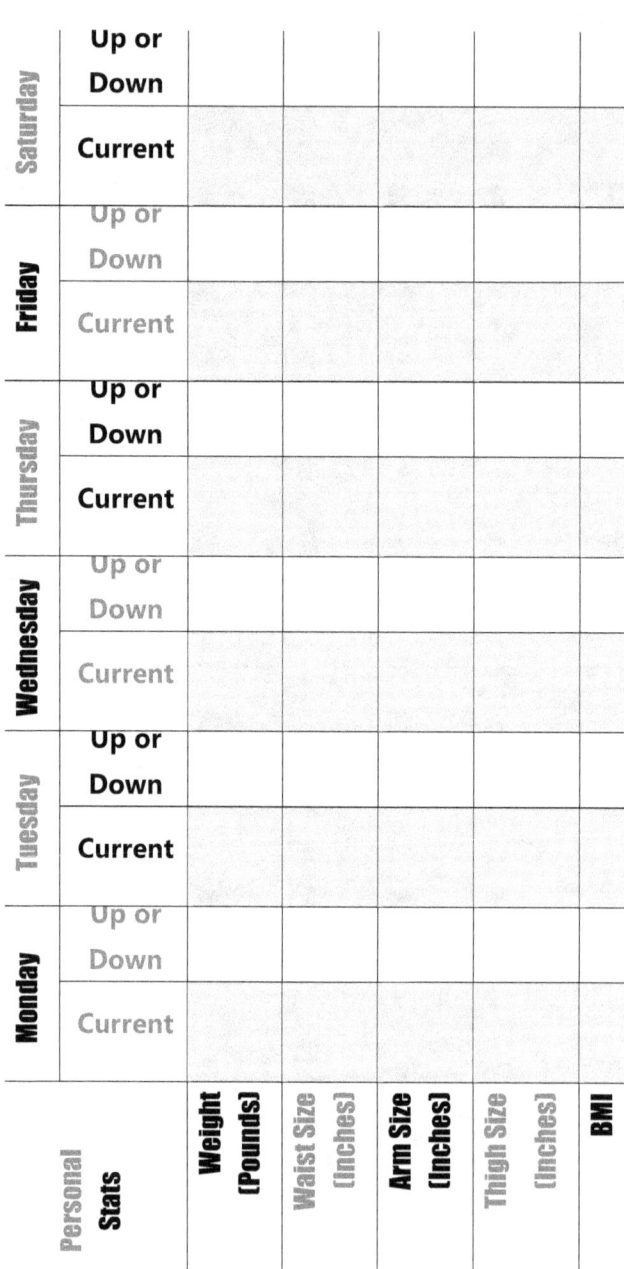

Progress Chart—Week 6

Personal Stats	Monday		Tuesday		Wednesday		Thursday		Friday		Saturday	
	Current	Up or Down	Current	Up or Down	Current	Up or Down	Current	Up or Down	Current	Up or Down	Current	Up or Down
Weight [Pounds]												
Waist Size [Inches]												
Arm Size [Inches]												
Thigh Size [Inches]												
BMI												

BMI Calculation

$$BMI = \frac{(\text{Weight in pounds} \times 703)}{(\text{Height in Inches} \times \text{Height in Inches})}$$

If you are unsure about working out any of these statistics then please refer to the main guide book which will explain these to you in more detail and help you to understand it better. Remember, you are doing well, keep it up.

Exercise Resolution
By Andrew Banks

Progress Chart—Week 7

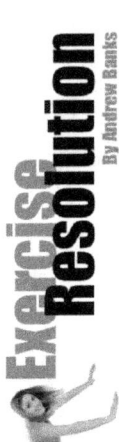

Exercise	Monday Required	Monday Complete?	Tuesday Required	Tuesday Complete?	Wednesday Required	Wednesday Complete?	Thursday Required	Thursday Complete?	Friday Required	Friday Complete?	Saturday Required	Saturday Complete?	Total
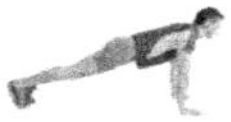 Push Ups	10	☐	10	☐	10	☐	10	☐	10	☐	10	☐	
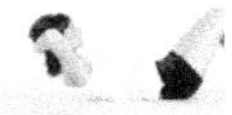 Sit Ups	10	☐	10	☐	10	☐	10	☐	10	☐	10	☐	
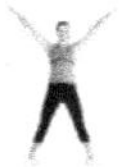 Star Jumps	25	☐	25	☐	30	☐	30	☐	30	☐	30	☐	
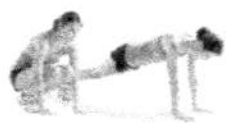 Squat Thrusts	10	☐	10	☐	10	☐	10	☐	10	☐	10	☐	
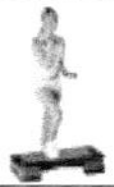 Step Ups	30	☐	30	☐	30	☐	30	☐	30	☐	30	☐	
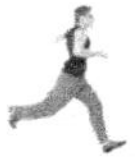 Run / Jog	2 mins	☐	2 mins	☐	2 mins	☐	2 mins	☐	2 mins	☐	2 mins	☐	

Exercise Resolution
By Andrew Banks

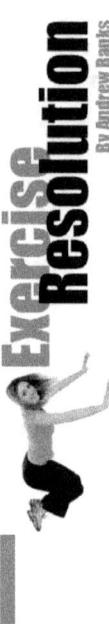

Progress Chart—Week 7

Personal Stats	Monday		Tuesday		Wednesday		Thursday		Friday		Saturday	
	Current	Up or Down	Current	Up or Down	Current	Up or Down	Current	Up or Down	Current	Up or Down	Current	Up or Down
Weight [Pounds]												
Waist Size [Inches]												
Arm Size [Inches]												
Thigh Size [Inches]												
BMI												

BMI Calculation

$$BMI = \frac{(\text{Weight in pounds} \times 703)}{(\text{Height in Inches} \times \text{Height in Inches})}$$

If you are unsure about working out any of these statistics then please refer to the main guide book which will explain these to you in more detail and help you to understand it better. Remember, you are doing well, keep it up.

Exercise Resolution
By Andrew Banks

Progress Chart—Week 8

Exercise	Monday Required	Monday Complete?	Tuesday Required	Tuesday Complete?	Wednesday Required	Wednesday Complete?	Thursday Required	Thursday Complete?	Friday Required	Friday Complete?	Saturday Required	Saturday Complete?	Total
Push Ups	10	☐	10	☐	10	☐	10	☐	10	☐	10	☐	
Sit Ups	10	☐	10	☐	10	☐	10	☐	10	☐	10	☐	
Star Jumps	30	☐	30	☐	30	☐	30	☐	30	☐	30	☐	
Squat Thrusts	10	☐	10	☐	10	☐	10	☐	10	☐	10	☐	
Step Ups	30	☐	30	☐	30	☐	30	☐	30	☐	30	☐	
Run / Jog	2 mins	☐	2 mins	☐	2 mins	☐	2 mins	☐	2 mins	☐	2 mins	☐	

Exercise Resolution
By Andrew Banks

Progress Chart—Week 8

Personal Stats	Monday Current	Monday Up or Down	Tuesday Current	Tuesday Up or Down	Wednesday Current	Wednesday Up or Down	Thursday Current	Thursday Up or Down	Friday Current	Friday Up or Down	Saturday Current	Saturday Up or Down
Weight [Pounds]												
Waist Size [Inches]												
Arm Size [Inches]												
Thigh Size [Inches]												
BMI												

BMI Calculation

$$BMI = \frac{(Weight\ in\ pounds \times 703)}{(Height\ in\ Inches \times Height\ in\ Inches)}$$

If you are unsure about working out any of these statistics then please refer to the main guide book which will explain these to you in more detail and help you to understand it better. Remember, you are doing well, keep it up.

Exercise Resolution
By Andrew Banks

Progress Chart—Week 9

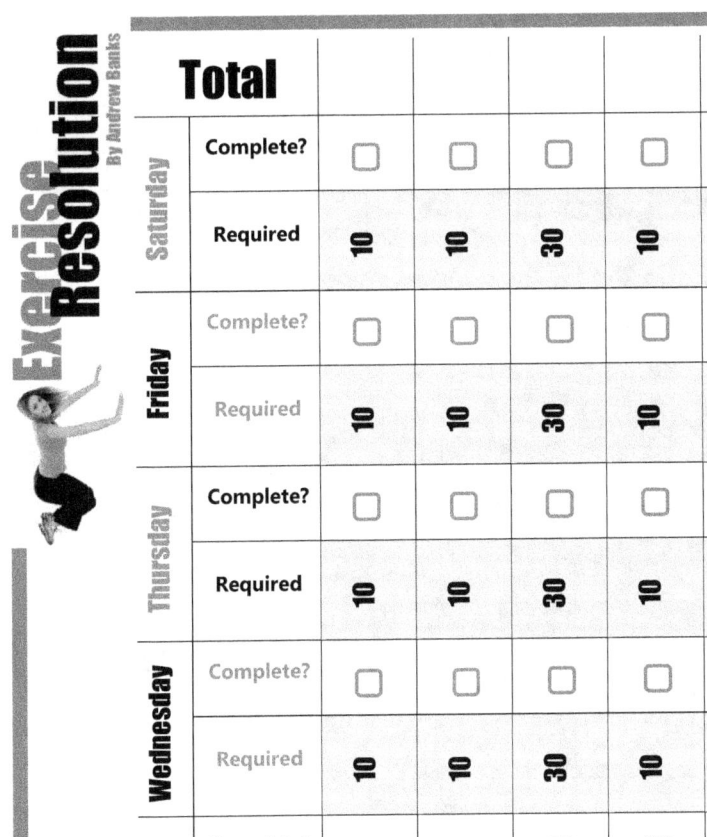

Exercise	Monday Required	Monday Complete?	Tuesday Required	Tuesday Complete?	Wednesday Required	Wednesday Complete?	Thursday Required	Thursday Complete?	Friday Required	Friday Complete?	Saturday Required	Saturday Complete?	Total
Push Ups	10	☐	10	☐	10	☐	10	☐	10	☐	10	☐	
Sit Ups	10	☐	10	☐	10	☐	10	☐	10	☐	10	☐	
Star Jumps	30	☐	30	☐	30	☐	30	☐	30	☐	30	☐	
Squat Thrusts	10	☐	10	☐	10	☐	10	☐	10	☐	10	☐	
Step Ups	30	☐	30	☐	30	☐	30	☐	30	☐	30	☐	
Run / Jog	2 mins	☐	2 mins	☐	2 mins	☐	2 mins	☐	2 mins	☐	2 mins	☐	

Exercise Resolution
By Andrew Banks

Progress Chart—Week 9

Personal Stats	Monday Current	Monday Up or Down	Tuesday Current	Tuesday Up or Down	Wednesday Current	Wednesday Up or Down	Thursday Current	Thursday Up or Down	Friday Current	Friday Up or Down	Saturday Current	Saturday Up or Down
Weight [Pounds]												
Waist Size [Inches]												
Arm Size [Inches]												
Thigh Size [Inches]												
BMI												

BMI Calculation

$$BMI = \frac{(Weight\ in\ pounds \times 703\ )}{(Height\ in\ Inches \times Height\ in\ Inches)}$$

If you are unsure about working out any of these statistics then please refer to the main guide book which will explain these to you in more detail and help you to understand it better. Remember, you are doing well, keep it up.

Progress Chart—Week ___

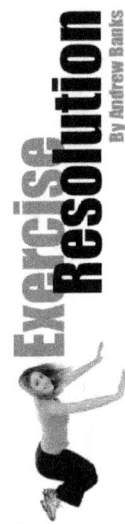

Exercise Resolution
By Andrew Banks

Exercise	Monday		Tuesday		Wednesday		Thursday		Friday		Saturday		Total
	Required	Complete?	Required	Complete?	Required	Complete?	Required	Complete?	Required	Complete?	Required	Complete?	
Push Ups		☐		☐		☐		☐		☐		☐	
Sit Ups		☐		☐		☐		☐		☐		☐	
Star Jumps		☐		☐		☐		☐		☐		☐	
Squat Thrusts		☐		☐		☐		☐		☐		☐	
Step Ups		☐		☐		☐		☐		☐		☐	
Run / Jog		☐		☐		☐		☐		☐		☐	

Exercise Resolution
By Andrew Banks

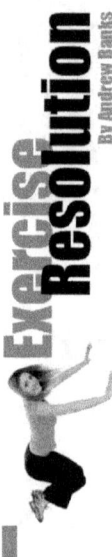

Progress Chart—Week _____

Personal Stats	Monday Current	Monday Up or Down	Tuesday Current	Tuesday Up or Down	Wednesday Current	Wednesday Up or Down	Thursday Current	Thursday Up or Down	Friday Current	Friday Up or Down	Saturday Current	Saturday Up or Down
Weight [Pounds]												
Waist Size [Inches]												
Arm Size [Inches]												
Thigh Size [Inches]												
BMI												

BMI Calculation

$$BMI = \frac{(\text{Weight in pounds} \times 703)}{(\text{Height in Inches} \times \text{Height in Inches})}$$

If you are unsure about working out any of these statistics then please refer to the main guide book which will explain these to you in more detail and help you to understand it better. Remember, you are doing well, keep it up.

Exercise Resolution
By Andrew Banks

Progress Chart—Personal Targets

Exercise	Week 31 Required	Week 31 Complete?	Week 32 Required	Week 32 Complete?	Week 33 Required	Week 33 Complete?	Week 34 Required	Week 34 Complete?	Week 35 Required	Week 35 Complete?	Week 36 Required	Week 36 Complete?
Push Ups		☐		☐		☐		☐		☐		☐
Sit Ups		☐		☐		☐		☐		☐		☐
Star Jumps		☐		☐		☐		☐		☐		☐
Squat Thrusts		☐		☐		☐		☐		☐		☐
Step Ups		☐		☐		☐		☐		☐		☐
Run / Jog		☐		☐		☐		☐		☐		☐

Progress Chart—Personal Targets

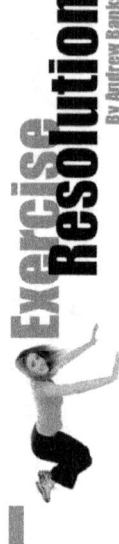

Exercise	Week 37		Week 38		Week 39		Week 40		Week 41		Week 42	
	Required	Complete?	Required	Complete?	Required	Complete?	Required	Complete?	Required	Complete?	Required	Complete?
Push Ups		☐		☐		☐		☐		☐		☐
Sit Ups		☐		☐		☐		☐		☐		☐
Star Jumps		☐		☐		☐		☐		☐		☐
Squat Thrusts		☐		☐		☐		☐		☐		☐
Step Ups		☐		☐		☐		☐		☐		☐
Run / Jog		☐		☐		☐		☐		☐		☐

Exercise Resolution

By Andrew Banks

Progress Chart—Personal Targets

Exercise	Week 43 Required	Week 43 Complete?	Week 44 Required	Week 44 Complete?	Week 45 Required	Week 45 Complete?	Week 46 Required	Week 46 Complete?	Week 47 Required	Week 47 Complete?	Week 48 Required	Week 48 Complete?
Push Ups		☐		☐		☐		☐		☐		☐
Sit Ups		☐		☐		☐		☐		☐		☐
Star Jumps		☐		☐		☐		☐		☐		☐
Squat Thrusts		☐		☐		☐		☐		☐		☐
Step Ups		☐		☐		☐		☐		☐		☐
Run / Jog		☐		☐		☐		☐		☐		☐

Progress Chart—Personal Targets

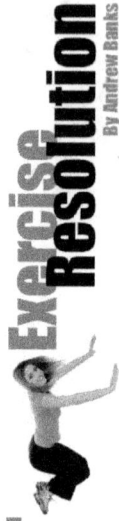

Exercise	Week 49 Required	Week 49 Complete?	Week 50 Required	Week 50 Complete?	Week 51 Required	Week 51 Complete?	Week 52 Required	Week 52 Complete?	Required	Complete?	Required	Complete?
Push Ups		☐		☐		☐		☐		☐		☐
Sit Ups		☐		☐		☐		☐		☐		☐
Star Jumps		☐		☐		☐		☐		☐		☐
Squat Thrusts		☐		☐		☐		☐		☐		☐
Step Ups		☐		☐		☐		☐		☐		☐
Run / Jog		☐		☐		☐		☐		☐		☐

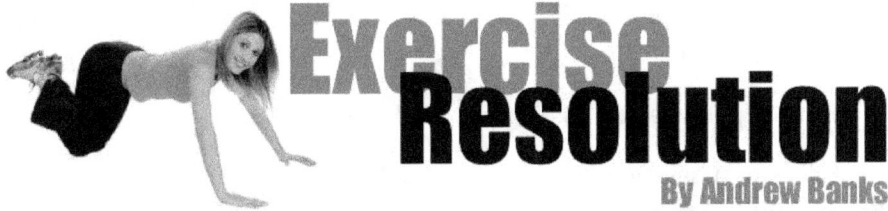

Exercise Resolution

By Andrew Banks

About the Author

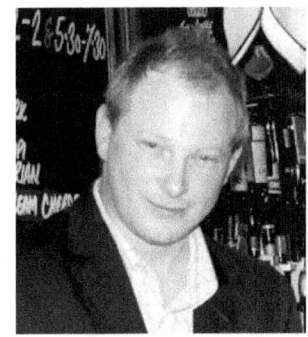

Andrew Banks is a man who has been working in the fitness and self-defence field for over 20 years now. Holding a 3rd Dan Black Belt in Wado-Ryu Based Karate and running Koku-Ryu Karate based in North Lincolnshire has helped him to challenge and channel his knowledge to individuals and groups for a long period of time.

Even though Andrew's main expertise is in Martial Arts, a main element of this is the development of fitness and health for students. This is due to the nature of Karate training and its physical requirements. Over the years Andrew has developed a list of skills in this area which have helped stretch and diversify his own training and help people become fitter and healthier.

This programme was developed by Andrew as a way of helping people who cannot afford the common run of the mill diet fads and gym memberships. After spending years hearing people wish they could be fit and spending money week in week out on diet programmes and gym memberships he decided that he would put his knowledge together in a simple, easy to use system that people could do from the comfort of their own homes with little cost.

How often have you wished you could lose weight?

How often have you wished you could get a little fitter?

How often have you wanted to have a healthier approach to life?

And how often have you thought I wish it was a lot cheaper?

The Exercise Resolution has the answer to all those questions. A low cost effective way to get fitter, healthier and does not require you to dig deep in your pockets.

All you need is you, that is it, just you and 5-10 minutes of your time. So go on....**give it a try!**

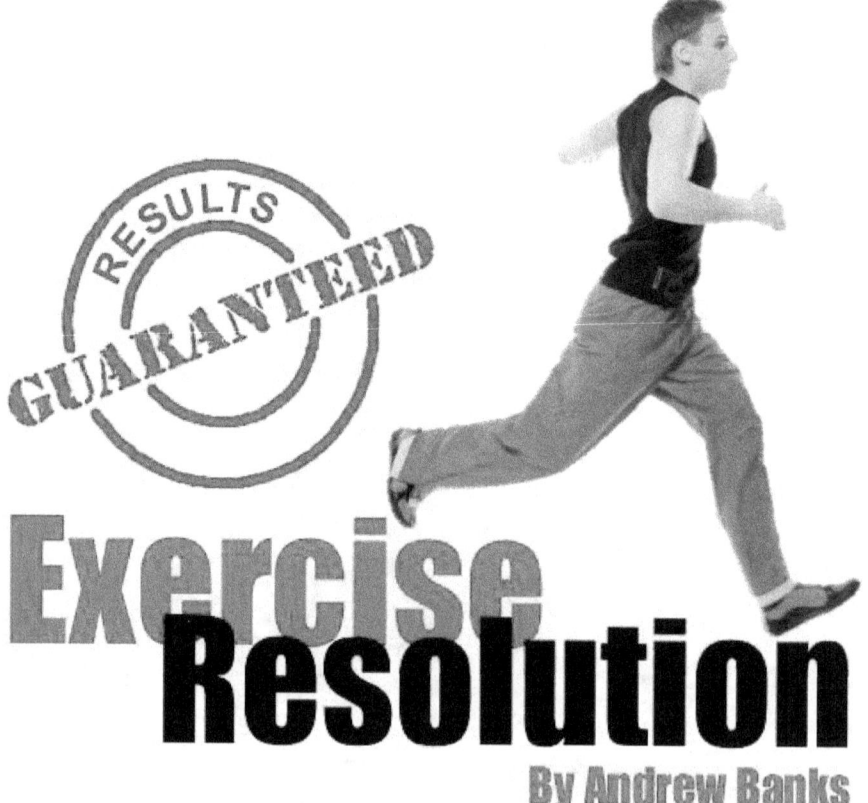

RESULTS GUARANTEED

Exercise Resolution

By Andrew Banks

www.ingramcontent.com/pod-product-compliance
Lightning Source LLC
Chambersburg PA
CBHW060154290526
45789CB00003B/1033